Eat It All Up

Getting Your Children to Eat What You Give Them (Not Just What They Want)

Louise Brennan

2012

CONTENTS

ACKNOWLEDGMENTS

Thanks to Mum for many creative ideas, to Roz for nutritional advice and positive reinforcement, to David for making me come back to the project many times and to Amanda, Emma-Jane and Suzy for editorial and other comments.

For Dad.

INTRODUCTION

My husband is a very successful man. He is the Managing Director of a large UK subsidiary of a global company. He has three happy healthy children and is himself healthy and fit. His favourite pastimes are travelling, walking, wine-tasting and following his football team. But there is one thing that quite significantly affects his quality of life. Occasionally we go out for a meal at a good restaurant. The type of restaurant that will only have about eight or nine choices of meal on the menu. And he will not be able to find a main course, starter or pudding that he looks forward to eating or really wants to eat. Sometimes he goes out to lunch with work colleagues or to conference-style events or gala dinners and he can't always face eating the food that is put in front of him, while everyone else round the table tucks in to theirs. If he goes to the sandwich shop during work, he knows what foods are healthy and good for him, but he can't find anything in that category that he actually likes to eat, so he has to choose whether to enjoy his lunch and feel guilty about what he eats, or not enjoy it while feeling more virtuous.

He is not a vegetarian and has no food allergies that we know of. It is just that there are so many things that he dislikes eating. As a child, he would not eat fruit and vegetables and was a "fussy" eater. He ate peas and carrots and liked chicken and roast potatoes. He ate puddings, cakes and biscuits and sugary drinks like lemonade. He didn't eat beef or celery, tomatoes, pasta, sweetcorn, marmite, cheese, cream. In fact, the things that he did like were a much shorter, easier list to draw up than the food he wouldn't eat.

My husband's quality of life is significantly affected by the limited range of foods that he enjoys eating. He doesn't always find eating out a relaxing and enjoyable experience. He can find going to friends' houses embarrassing when he is unable to eat what he is offered by them. He struggles to maintain a healthy diet, because how do you manage to eat five portions of fruit and vegetables each day, if you don't actually like the fruit or vegetables on offer?

When our children were born, we agreed that this was a reality of his life but it did not need to be part of theirs. They have been brought up from the start to eat everything and to enjoy food. They have been taken to cafes and restaurants since they were tiny babies. They can be trusted to sit still, be fairly quiet and polite and to eat a proper meal from the main menu. They know that they are allowed to eat cakes and sweets, but not all the time and not if they haven't eaten their main meal and healthy foods. They do not argue with us at mealtimes and they don't try and negotiate snacks and sweets. They enjoy helping with cooking and the social activity of eating meals as a family. They sometimes discuss food and what they might be eating at their next meal. While having their own ideas about what they like or do not like, they are willing to try any food and make their own judgement of its merits.

As an adult, my husband's tastes have gradually broadened. In part, this is because he is married to a food dictator with very diverse tastes in food. He has also put a lot of effort into trying new foods and building relationships with vegetables, fish and meat that had never been introduced to him previously. He now likes beetroot, celeriac salad, lamb chops, mussels and even grapefruit.

This book is for all of you who want your children to grow up to be able to choose anything whatsoever from the menu. For those of you who want your children to really enjoy food and eating it. And it is for those of you who know what healthy food is and who want your children to make the best possible diet choices of their own for a healthy future. It is for you if you are starting to be concerned about whether your child is eating enough of the right kinds of food, or if they are becoming "picky" and refusing to eat various things. It is also for you if you find the whole process of cooking and having meals with your family far too difficult and stressful. If eating as a family is not an enjoyable experience then you need to read this book. If your teenagers are refusing to eat with you at all this book is also for you.

Of course, this book is for my husband as well. He has worked so hard to balance his own needs with those of his children and, in doing so, has learned to enjoy many things which he previously detested.

The aim of this book is to help you to get the children of your family to eat everything that they are given. What I have set out in the chapters and pages that follow are a series of clear and simple rules which will encourage your child or children to eat the broadest range of food possible. The approach is divided into two main sections – one for very little children, from when they first start to eat solid foods, and one for older children whose eating habits may already be causing problems. Each rule is supported with an explanation and ideas for following it through. Often, I provide a rationale based upon well-understood approaches to the development of children. There are also plenty of stories and real-life examples which will help you to understand the reasons why children can fall into bad habits and what you can do about them.

Why is it important not to let your children establish bad eating habits? Well, it really is true that *what you eat as a child influences what you eat for the rest of your life*. This means that if much of your diet between the ages of about six months and sixteen years is based on white bread, pizza bases, white pasta, red and poor quality meat, biscuits, sugary drinks and so forth, you will include these as the main part of your adult diet. It will be much harder to kick the habit of eating these essentially low-health foods, even though you will know that fruit, vegetables, fish, pulses and wholemeal options are better for you.

And why is it so important to get your children to eat everything? Because if they are happy to eat broccoli, carrots, celeriac, mackerel, raspberries, bulgar wheat, porridge and cashew nuts *as well as* chocolate cake, fromage frais and bacon sandwiches, they will be able to choose those healthy foods when they need to in order to keep themselves in good shape - hopefully, for a long life. But if your child grows up always preferring cake, fromage frais and bacon and hardly ever eats broccoli and all those other good things, they will tend to crave the choice of the bacon or the cake when they are an adult. And that can lead to a life of less-than-optimum health, guilt-laden meal and snack choices and probably crash- and other inappropriate forms of dieting. Dieting already makes life a misery for far too many of us – why inflict this cycle on our children?

It is worth mentioning here, although it is stating the obvious, that people who become overweight are more likely to suffer from illnesses which range from those affecting quality-of-life to those which are actually life-threatening. I dwell in slightly more detail on this early in the book. But being overweight and generally unhealthy will affect life-chances and psychological well-being, too.

I'll bet that you do not want to spend any more time than you have to worrying about what your children will eat today and whether it will influence their future health and well-being. You probably have more than enough to think about – work, washing, school clubs, Christmas coming up, new shoes to buy the toddler, paying for a school trip. The less energy and time you spend arguing with the children about what they are going to have for tea, the better it will be all round. And that may be why many families get into the situation of giving in to "picky" eaters, children who want junk food and no vegetables on their plate. Because, quite frankly, it is easier to let it be than to tackle the problem. But if you are determined to start on the right track or to bring everyone back to it, then you *will* find that you spend less time on the issue overall. Because you will be able to pick anything from your personal repertoire of meals to cook or prepare, safe in the knowledge that everyone in the house will sit down with you and eat it without complaining.

How to read this book

This is not a long, complicated book, because I want you to see and understand that getting your children to eat a balanced healthy diet is a relatively straightforward process.

I don't want you to feel like a "bad" parent if your child or children are already starting to be picky or fussy about food. The fact that you are reading this book means that you want to support and help your child and your whole family (including yourself) and I really hope that it will provide many practical ways in which you can do this.

In Chapter one I outline what many children do eat today and why, for many, this will affect their health, their life-expectancy and their life-chances.

Chapter 2 sets out briefly the pressure on parents and why it can be so hard to respond to the bombardment of conflicting information and advice we are given, including the facts about food allergies.

In Chapter 3 I have provided a series of key rules which will help all parents. This chapter is headed as "for the very young", but many of the principles and guidelines that I describe can be applied to any age of child. So if your six-year-old is a very fussy eater, you will find this chapter as useful as those later in the book.

Chapter 4 emphasises some principles behind the thinking in Chapter 3. It will help you to rationalise some of the behaviours of your children. It talks about your role as a parent and also provides some context around real concerns which parents have.

Chapter 5 is for parents of children from the age of about four or five up to teenagers. Building on the ideas from Chapter 3, it applies these to the older child and gives some ideas of how you can work together as a family to tackle issues relating to food and eating. It introduces the idea of using a food diary and reward charts to improve the eating habits of your family.

Chapter 6 provides some background nutritional information which will help if you do not feel confident about exactly what your children should be eating. The nutritional advice in this book has been independently checked and approved by a clinical nutritionist.

Find out more

The aim of "Eat It All Up" is to give you the confidence and knowledge to support positive eating behaviours in your children and the whole family.

There are references in the book to a variety of useful websites which can guide you through issues such as how to put together a healthy meal, the likelihood that eating problems are linked to allergies and so on – you'll see these as you read through.

If you want to find out more, get in touch with an expert or ask a specific question about something you read here, please try my website:

www.eatitallup.com

Or go to my Twitter page:

@louiseeatsitall

1 WHY IT MATTERS WHAT OUR CHILDREN EAT

I hope you are feeling relaxed and positive because this first chapter of the book is going to outline some pretty scary statistics about diet and eating in the UK. Many of the trends are global – in the US, obesity is becoming a national crisis and even in countries with "good" diets, such as Japan and Mediterranean nations, food choices and habits of eating are gradually becoming less healthy. This is why it is important that your children eat what you give them and that what you give them is worth eating.

I think there has been so much media attention on the role of diet on the health of the UK population that it is unnecessary for me to cover this in much detail. You already know that you and your family should be eating five portions of fruit and vegetables per day (more if you are reading this in the US.) Nevertheless, I have highlighted some key points and statistics in this chapter to heighten your level of awareness and remind you just how important it is for our offspring to get off to as good a start as possible in their lives. It is one thing reading about the diet of schoolchildren in a newspaper and quite another to understand what organizations such as the British Medical Association have to say about it.

What children eat – and don't eat

Here is a story.

Once there was a little boy called "John" and by the time he was two years old, he mostly ate jam sandwiches. He ate jam sandwiches for breakfast, lunch, tea and supper and when he wanted a snack he ate biscuits. His parents took him to the doctor to explain that John only ate jam sandwiches and the doctor said "Don't worry - he seems to be healthy enough and I am sure he will eat more things as he gets older." So John's Mum and Dad took him home and life went on as before. The doctor was right, of course - John did eat more things as he got older. In fact, when I last saw John he was a thriving nine year old and for his lunch that day he ate a plate of chips and drank a can of cola. For pudding, he tried jam roly-poly, but he didn't like it and left it on his plate.

This is actually a true story about a child I know and, you may have a similar anecdote of your own that you could tell. Even if you exclude this extreme example, many children start off with unhealthy diets and continue with these habits into their teenage years and on into adulthood. When I talk about an unhealthy diet, I mean one that is:

Limited in the range of food eaten; low in key nutritional groups; high in "poor" foods, such as those containing a lot of sugars, salt and fats and reliant on processed food.

"Why," you may ask, "Are these children not unhealthy – suffering from malnutrition or other disorders?" The reason is the opposite of malnutrition – it is a phenomenon called over-nourishment. Basically, in the UK and many other countries today, children's (and adults') diets have far higher levels of carbohydrates and proteins than they did in the past. Think, for example, of how much meat we generally eat. In previous centuries and even decades, meat was eaten once or twice each week. Now, it is acceptable to eat meat almost at every meal on every day – bacon for breakfast, chicken sandwich at lunchtime and shepherd's pie for dinner. This means that children grow quickly, becoming larger than they used to, but without necessarily consuming the right balance of foods.

There is more about what children should eat and specific issues relating to food preparation, cooking and ingredients in chapter 6.

An unhealthy diet is different from a poor diet. A poor diet is caused by a lack of money or essential resources to feed a family. If a child from, say, Malawi starts off in life with a poor diet and is then adopted by a western family, he or she is likely to be taller and healthier in the long-term than a friend who continues to live in their original early environment[i]. There is no contention that a good diet is better for a growing child than a poor one. Unfortunately, in our more "affluent" society, we appear to have crawled straight through the small window of healthy eating and to be coming out the other side. Whereas our education and means should result in better nutrition standards for everyone, it seems that how and what we choose to eat is making our health worse. It is only recently that society seems to have noticed what is going on.

The impact of what we eat

On average, more than half of us are fatter than we should be. In England the number of people who are overweight and classified as clinically obese has been rising rapidly. In 2009 61.3% of adults and 28.3% of children aged between two and ten were overweight or obese and, of those, 23% of adults and 14.4% of children were obese[ii].

Amazingly, even though most of us now have more money for food and more information about food than ever before, our children do not seem to eating the right things.

The most recent study by the Department of Health to assess the nutritional status of the nation found that children on average consumed more sugar than they should – the main contributor being soft drinks. They also ate fewer than the five portions of vegetables recommended daily: for boys this was 3.1 portions per day and for girls only 2.7 portions[iii]. About 42% of children aged five eat less than three portions of fruit or vegetables each day and around 21.5% eat less than two portions daily[iv].

The Department of Health's website and the internet in general is peppered with statistics about diet and obesity. For example, one study found that most children ate a bag of crisps every day. This provides the nutritional equivalent of drinking a five litre bottle of vegetable oil each year[v] – yum. Many of the children in another survey ate sweets and/or chocolate every day[vi].

Dr Sam Everington, who supported the work of the BMA in producing the report "Preventing Childhood Obesity," stated that "Obesity and malnutrition is now a common presentation in the GP surgery. Over half my children patients are malnourished, many are obese."[vii]

The study itself went on to say "It is accepted that dietary patterns common in childhood, such as regular consumption of high-fat and sugar-containing foods and low fruit and vegetable intake, are associated with a poor diet later in life."[viii] The reason that this should concern all of us is that while adults are in control and can choose what they have to eat, the majority of children cannot. Not only do they not have the power of money within a family with which to buy foods, they are less able to control their basic impulses. In other words, until someone reaches a certain level of maturity, they have little chance of organizing a healthy diet for themselves.

So to recap, the research says that what a child eats when it is young affects what it eats for the rest of its life. And the people who set and establish those dietary patterns are the parents, grand-parents and all other carers of your child. When your children are small, most of what they eat is controlled not by themselves, but by others. And, in fact, research done with obese children shows that when families are all involved in programmes to help them lose weight, the children lose weight faster and stay a healthier weight then those who are on individual programmes[ix].

Here is a story about role models.

When I went to my child's nursery one day, there was a big notice attached to the door. It said,

"Please provide a sunhat and cream for your child now the days are getting brighter. Any child who does not have a hat and cream will not be allowed to play outside."

A few days later I went to pick my daughter up from the nursery. The children were playing outside and most of them were wearing hats. But not one of their carers had a hat on. Surely, if we ask a child to put on a hat for health reasons, then we should be leading by example and demonstrating that we also accept the message that over-exposure to the sun is dangerous. Why give the message that protecting your health is something that you only do as a child - not as an adult?

I think that many parents do a similar thing to this with food – but the other way round: how often have you seen Mum or Dad tucking into a healthy salad or bowl of vegetable soup while their children are sitting there with a cardboard box containing a white ham sandwich, packet of crisps and carton of sugary drink, or a plate of "chicken dippers" and chips? Do these parents live with the strange belief that, while they need to look after their own bodies, their children are not important and therefore they do not have to look after theirs?

Joanna Blythman, who has researched the eating and mealtime habits of the British people, lists a related attitude as one of Britain's "top ten bad food beliefs." She says that what we think is the following: "There is no point in giving children good food. They won't appreciate it."[x] I don't believe this to be true – many children are very discerning about what they eat and can learn to choose and enjoy good food from a young age. What is more, I think that what a child eats is the most important thing determining their future health and well-being. So, what *you* choose to feed your children, or what you choose to let them eat, will play a big part in deciding how healthy and happy they are as they get older *and* as adults.

Linking major illnesses and diet

The links between cancer and what we eat are now widely reported. The amazing EPIC study, which is following the diet and cancer incidence of over half a million people across Europe, has already come up with some clear indications regarding cancer and diet in a number of areas. Examples are:

- They have identified that eating a lot of fibre-rich food reduces the risk of bowel cancer
- Eating large quantities of red or processed meat is linked to the incidence of bowel, stomach and pancreatic cancers
- Being overweight increases the risk of getting certain cancers
- Eating lots of fruit and vegetables has wide health benefits, including reduced incidence of mouth, oesophageal and lung cancers.

The EPIC study can be accessed via the Cancer Research UK website.

Research is filling in more and more of the information around what exactly is a health-giving diet – rather than illness-causing. The Department of Health recently stated that, after reducing smoking, eating more fruit and vegetables may be the most effective cancer prevention strategy[xi]. Cancer Research UK's advice is to eat a diet high in fibre, fruit and vegetables and low in red and processed meat, saturated fat and salt.

Eating a diet high in fruit and vegetables is also thought to reduce the chances and severity of asthma attacks according to research reported by Asthma UK[xii]. Conversely, being overweight increases risks of coronary heart disease and strokes. The key risk factors for these illnesses are physical inactivity, obesity and smoking. Having diabetes also increases risk.

Type 2 diabetes is also known as "adult onset" diabetes because, until now, it has rarely been found in children. However, the rates of this type of diabetes are rising rapidly – both for children, teenagers and grown-ups. The illness is related to what you eat, whether you are overweight and how much exercise you do. The British Medical Association describes the increasing number of children with type 2 diabetes as "a particularly alarming consequence of the obesity epidemic."[xiii] Diabetes itself leads to the likelihood of other serious diseases, including cardiovascular disease (CHD and strokes), kidney failure, loss of sight and amputations and the younger you are when you first get the illness, the more likely it is that one or more of these consequences will occur[xiv]. Obesity is the greatest risk factor for the onset of diabetes in childhood.

It should be remembered that all of the conditions I have mentioned above reduce life expectancy significantly.

Sadly, overweight people often experience problems in social and emotional aspects of their development. Children will initially choose friends based on how attractive they think they are. Overweight children are seen as less likeable than those with a physical disability. This finding was first reported in 1961 and repeated in 2001. The researchers found that stigmatisation of obese children had increased in the 40 year gap[xv]. In the longer term, overweight people suffer ongoing discrimination and have fewer positive life chances than their thinner counterparts – they have lower incomes overall and are less likely to get married, for example[xvi]. They are found to have lower aspirations and overall satisfaction with their life.

Summary

We are seeing the results of a gradual deterioration of the way in which British people eat and of their attitude to food and exercise. This is obvious in the health and weight of many children in society. And in the long term, this will cost us – overweight and obese children will have unhealthy, shorter lives to look forward to. They may live for many years with debilitating, painful illnesses, which dramatically reduce the quality of their life. Through their lifetimes, they will cost the taxpayer more money. And their lives are likely to be less fulfilling and happy than they should be.

The Government has responded by setting some very clear standards for food in schools. But it is unlikely to exert much pressure on the food industry and especially on the powerful snack- and fast-food companies which encourage the unhealthy eating habits which are linked to the increasing numbers of overweight and obese people. And it is also starting to make it clear that much of the responsibility for how our children eat is down to us as parents.

I think the best summary for this chapter comes from the mouth of Jamie Oliver, quoted during his campaign to improve school meals in 2004[xvii]. "The other really important thing is making people understand. People say "My kid eats this or that junk food and he's all right." They don't realise what the long-term effect's gonna be. It takes a doctor or paediatrician to say to them, your kid's storing up this that or the other health problem. The information's all there: the statistics show that we're growing more obese, getting more diseases linked with poor diet. We should be saying, f--- it, what are we doing? If we don't act now, in 100 years what will people think – they'll look back and see, all the signs were there – and they'll say why didn't they do something?"

He is right. We know what we should be doing and there is no excuse for not making sure our children eat properly and healthily. The rules I have set out to help you get your child to eat the food you give them will ensure that he or she is not a future victim of poor food and lifestyle choices.

2 DON'T PANIC – I'M A PARENT

How did we get here?

I think there is a kind of mental programming that society inflicts upon many mothers and fathers of young children. This results in a number of factors that come together in generating a sense of anxiety and concern about children and food. The first of these is what I call the "myth of children's food." This is the idea that babies and young children, in particular, are only supposed to like and want to eat bland-tasting, easy-to-chew foods. So, for example, when I went to a child's first birthday party recently, I noticed that all the adults were eating salad, bread, meat, cheese and that there was fruit salad for pudding. But the one-year-old had a plate of buttered white bread, cheese chunks and ham, with some grapes. These had all been selected from the main buffet. And they weren't nearly as interesting or varied as some of the other things that were on offer. I think that many parents do this to make sure that at least something is eaten. But the outcome will be that the child will get used to always eating the limited range of food, textures and tastes and will then find it less enticing to try other things over time. The end-point is the ubiquitous "children's menu" which is now so common. And most of us could dictate that menu from memory – "Pasta with tomato sauce, beefburger, chips and peas, fishfingers, chips and peas".... and so on. Even if you opt for the "healthier" versions of these tried-and-tested favourites, you are still encouraging your child to limit his or her choices of food to elements which are, generally, less healthy than lots of other things they could be eating.

I think there is another example of "brain-washing" for parents. It is the idea that children, for some reason, are *supposed* to be fussy about food.

In much of the world, children have subsistence diets which consist of a basic starchy-carbohydrate – rice, yam, bread or similar – and often nothing else. They eat this every day of their lives. They get protein maybe once or twice a week, sometimes less. They are not going to be fussy about the odd fish curry or bean stew that comes their way: they are going to eat it. Our children are not programmed to be fussy. They are lively, active and sometimes challenging. Being "difficult" about some choices in their lives is normal. Being a bit funny about food is just one of many things they do. You wouldn't ignore or accept it if your child decided to let go of your hand and run across the road every time you walked them to school – I expect you would make a clear rule or have a strategy for managing this. Why do many of us not have a similar strategy or set of rules for getting their children to eat well?

The third way in which I believe that parents are brow-beaten by society is just the general pressure to feed our children the right foods and to make sure they *are* healthy. I vividly remember feeling anxious if one of my little ones seemed not to be eating well. I recall worrying about the fact that one or other of them had not had much fruit today, or that they had only had a small tea and this might not get them through the night. I have no idea what drove these concerns, but they were real and I found them stressful. I am sure that I am not alone in feeling that I had to do the best to make sure my children ate well and that this developed something close to fear that I was not doing the right thing.

Jamie Oliver

Whatever your personal opinion on Jamie Oliver, it would be hard to argue that he does not have a strong view on what children should eat. The fact that he was willing to present this articulately (albeit with the odd f-word thrown in) to the whole of the United Kingdom and to follow it up with a lot of very hard work in support of his campaign to make school meals healthy makes him, in my eyes, a national hero. It did make everyone start to think about what their children eat. There is no compromise with Jamie: our children are getting fatter and unhealthier and losing touch with what was the "normal" food of the past.

It is no accident that his manifesto for making the food our children eat healthier, barely mentioned the children themselves. This is because he understands that children only make healthy choices when they are encouraged or positioned to do so by adults. The elements of his manifesto were making cookery classes compulsory, training new cookery teachers, empowering head teachers to get rid of junk food in schools, investing in dinner ladies and educating parents. He also wanted a "long-term public campaign to get people back onto a proper diet and empower/persuade (and possibly scare, if needed) the public into making better choices." It is quite clear where Jamie thinks a lot of the responsibility lies. Not just with the Government, but with the adult population in general and with parents having a key role in turning things around. No wonder so many parents are starting to feel the grip of guilt and panic as they realise how big an issue what their children eat has become.

What children should be eating

What a mis-mash of confused messages! On the one hand, there is plenty of advice out there saying "don't worry, leave it alone, it will all come out right in the end" — even from health professionals - and on the other hand, experienced GPs and nutritionists are warning us that a huge proportion of children are not eating the right foods to satisfy their basic nutritional requirements. How can it be right to leave things alone, then?

Lots of people still seem to be struggling with the concept of a balanced diet. Some people in my own family think that potatoes are a vegetable, so please believe me when I say that I do understand anyone who says they are having difficulty getting the healthy food message out to their offspring. Nevertheless, you would have to have been living in another galaxy – or at least avoided television, radio and newspapers, not to mention the major supermarket chains - to have missed the general knowledge that exists these days around some aspects of this. Is there anyone you know who has not seen the "five-a-day" message around fruit and vegetables, for example? Yet, it seems from the various studies, that these messages are not being translated into what children eat.

I don't think, therefore, that this is about understanding diet and nutrition, it is about putting into practice what you know is the best thing to do. Children – especially young children - respond to simple messages. That is why "five-a-day" is good, because anyone can grasp what it means. At the end of every day, you can count up how many of the five have been consumed. If more have been eaten, bingo! As parents, the best we can do is to make sure we understand key food messages – wholemeal options, fresh fruit and vegetables, limited red and processed meat, a reasonable amount of fish and, there you go, there is no room left for the cakes and biscuits. It is all too easy to over-complicate the food and nutritional advice that is out there. There is plenty of it, after all!

Too much information?

Leaving the basic nutritional messages aside, however, there is a vast range of information and advice about what, how and why we should be eating certain things. With every season there comes a "new" food that will make our lives bouncier and fuller and give us back that always-needed sense of well-being. This week it could be beetroot, wild garlic, raw beef, grapefruit, black rice or some obscure nutritional supplement. My view is that many foods are good for health and can be part of a nutritionally-balanced diet. But that diet should involve the widest possible range of good foods, rather than concentrating on a few "super" foods that are supposed to meet every need of our bodies. I suggest we would all be better to avoid fads and just follow sensible eating patterns every day.

Then there are the "food scares" which alert us to potentially life-threatening components in everyday foods. I have been much more aware of this since having children myself.

At one point our health visitor said that we should not be giving prawns to the children (they were about three and eighteen months at the time) and I have to confess that it had never even occurred to me that there may be any issue about feeding them seafood. But when I checked on the Food Standards Agency website, the information there stated that shellfish allergy was most common in adults. In other words, there is no reason why a child should not be allowed to eat shellfish. This type of contradictory advice seems to be endemic in the media and among professionals. Is it any wonder, then, that parents are confused and frightened about what they should give their children?

Quite rightly we are also warned about the presence of potentially dangerous elements in our food. Well-publicised examples include the possibility in 2006 of contracting salmonella from certain Cadbury's chocolate bars,[xviii] the outbreak of BSE in cattle during the 1990s and the presence of banned food colourings Para Red and Sudan I in various spicy foods in 2005. But the media go further to fuel our fears by publishing shocking and extreme eating accidents - often these are of children or adults choking on otherwise innocuous types of food - grapes, boiled sweets, even a fry-up in a greasy spoon café, have all hit the headlines.

Other food "scares" focus on the presence of specific ingredients, such as aspartame, preservatives and colourings in food. Sometimes, these problems and concerns are evidenced by clear scientific findings. Often, however, they are not.

How are we supposed to keep up with all this information? My daughter suffers from asthma and eczema, so I just typed "sesame seeds eczema asthma" into my internet search engine: It came up with over 39,000 results. How can that amount of data be of any use to me as a lay-person? And how am I supposed to use that information to decide what type and range of food to feed my children? I think that common sense has to prevail. Because if you think about it, how many real issues have you come across relating to what your children or the children of friends are able to eat?

Fear about food allergies

Here is what the Food Standards Agency actually says about food allergies:

"A number of surveys have found that 20-30% of people claim to have a food allergy. However, a Food Standards Agency (FSA) report in 2008 estimated that only 5-8% of children and 1-2% of adults have a food allergy. Some researchers believe that the figure for adults may be slightly higher, at around 3-4%.

The reason why many people think they have a food allergy is that they mistake an intolerance to certain types of food (which does not involve the immune system) for a food allergy (which does)."[xix]

In children, the foods that most commonly cause an allergic reaction are:

- eggs
- milk
- soya
- wheat
- peanuts.

The FSA also notes that most children will 'outgrow' food allergies to milk, eggs, soya and wheat by the time that they start school, although allergies to peanuts generally persist through the child's life – this is the case for about 80% of children with a peanut allergy.

Taking the statistics a bit further, researchers identified deaths from food allergies as very few. In a ten year period, there were eight deaths. There are around thirteen million children in the United Kingdom.[xx]

Of course if you have any concerns about the way your child seems or behaves after food, then you should talk to your GP about it. They may advise you whether it would be useful to have testing which can identify food intolerances. But the point is that many reactions are normal or just part of the body's growing up process and the risks are much lower than the media would have us believe.

Preaching to the converted

I think that, for many of you, this chapter is a case of preaching to the converted. I suspect that the reason that you are actually reading the book is because you *know* what your child or children should be eating. You already know about fruit and vegetables and what a balanced diet contains. And you understand why it is important for children to be a healthy weight.

You might be reading the book because you do not feel confident about getting your child to eat the right foods and you don't know how to get them to eat what you know they should. Or, you have started to find that food choices in your house are being restricted because one or more "little people" are getting increasingly difficult to please. Your child may already be refusing all sorts of lovely healthy foods and only eating the things that you are trying to avoid – biscuits and cakes. And you just feel relieved that they are at least eating *something*. Or you have reached a point where you are offering them pasta, peas and carrots every day for tea, because you know they will eat it. And you may have started buying those dried fruit tubes wrapped in foil that you can get in the organics section of the supermarket, because you are at your wits' end about how to get your little boy or girl to eat fruit.

What you would like is for your child to choose to eat the healthy foods; to prefer a piece of fruit to a piece of cake and to be happy to eat everything they are given – whether they are at home, with Grandma or at a friend's house.

Summary

The outcome of all of these factors is parental panic. Not in the literal sense of mothers crying hysterically in the supermarket, but something more subtle. Faced with a choice between food that is familiar, satisfying and broadly understood to be "safe" and a food that is new, unknown in its taste and nutritional value and slightly out of the ordinary, what would you choose? And how does the information you have about food make you respond to making those choices on behalf of your children?

It is only human for us to want to limit the exposure of both ourselves and our children to potential harm and one way of doing this is by reducing the range of food that we offer our family. This approach to managing the range of food that people eat is illustrated by two more stories.

Our family met a large group of friends for lunch at a sea-food restaurant. All of us love fish. When the menus came, everyone decided to share three of the giant seafood platters that were on offer - crab, mussels, cockles, oysters and many other delights. Our children and the three other children who were there all ate whatever they wanted and, of course, when they ate the cockle or the oyster, they got to take the shells home with them! I believe that many parents would worry about whether or not their children should eat seafood at all, let alone as their main meal of the day.

At a party at our house, a friend asked me if he could move the olives, because their little girl had never had them before. Olives are salty and obviously too many of them are not a good idea for a small child. But not to let her even try one seemed a shame to me. Personally, I would rather my children ate a small bowl of olives than a small packet of crisps (and they didn't ask me to move those!)

Parents have become supremely unconfident about both what to feed their children and how to feed them.

They know that they should be aiming for a balanced diet and I think that they are all pretty clear about the five fruit and vegetables a day. But then they have all this other information and misinformation: these things which should be good are actually bad - nuts, cheese and seafood, for example; these other things which we thought were fine are potentially dangerous, such as salty foods; we shouldn't be giving them these things because they can cause allergies, and so on. So we start to get to a limited range of foods that Mum or Dad:

   a)   are happy to eat themselves
   b)   know how prepare and cook
   c)   are certain will do no harm
   d)   are certain that will be healthy.

Not many of us have a "perfect diet". I eat too many dairy products, especially cheese. But avoiding food of poor nutritional quality and eating food which is better for us does have results. My daughter regularly leaves cakes and biscuits on her plate, uneaten. These and other "unhealthy" foods are the only things I never insist she tries out. She really doesn't like them and I believe this is because we don't eat them often at home. She loves a good curry, but has hardly ever eaten chicken nuggets. She was given them once with chips and peas. She ate the peas and chips and, although we got her to try them, she left the nuggets.

Like many people, when my children were born, I made new friends who had babies of the same age. We spent time together in small and large groups and could all see the way in which the children developed and changed. Inevitably, close friendships are nurtured by similar attitudes to how children should be brought up. I noticed that many of the other Mums and Dads that we became most friendly with had the same ideas about bed-times, table manners, how much television should be watched and what children should eat. I also noticed that some children, like our own, ate almost everything. But other children started to limit what they ate from a very young age.

What was the difference between the children who ate everything and those who did not? Essentially, it boiled down to parental attitudes towards food choices and eating and how parents managed mealtimes. I realise that some people saw us as "stricter" parents. But our children enjoy food – all varieties of food – and they choose healthy things to eat. They are happy at mealtimes, when we all sit together and talk to each other. There is no stress, no worry about what will be for dinner – we know it will be fairly healthy, good to eat and everyone will enjoy eating it.

3 PRACTICAL ADVICE FOR THE VERY YOUNG

This chapter of the book aims to give you a clear framework for establishing good eating habits for very young children from the start of their first proper food experiences. I believe that this framework applies, with little modification, to almost any child, of whatever age.

It will also provide practical ideas and strategies for ensuring that your children choose, eat and enjoy the best possible range of food. Much of what you read will be intuitive. You will think "oh yes, that is obvious." While you may agree with much of what I write, you must at the same time ask yourself "Is this what I/we actually do or how I/we behave?" and "How would I/we apply this in practice?"

Your role

I believe that the most important factor in determining the food that your children will choose to eat is how their parents and other primary carers behave. If you find it hard to carry out the advice in this book (I hope that you do not,) it will be much, much harder if you yourself do not act as a good example to your children. You need to be three things if you are to succeed:

1) You must be an advocate for food – lovely, tasty, enjoyable, healthy food – at all times emphasising the importance of food in the life of your family.

2) You must be a positive role model. Be interested in food and new food, trying out different recipes and making the whole eating experience something associated with family enjoyment.

3) Finally, you must make sure that you provide healthy food at home and keep junk food to a minimum. There are some ideas to help you with this, if you need them, in chapter 6.

I have set out the advice as a series of rules, because I think these are easier to remember than an entire book's worth of information. Some people draw up a list of their key rules on a sheet of paper, which they put up in a place where everyone in the family can see it. This helps to avoid conflicts and confusion and ensures consistent application of what has been agreed. You know what happens when you and a partner disagree on any aspect of discipline or behaviour: just as importantly, you should maintain a united front on the issue of food and eating.

The primary rule, which covers all of the others and has to be applied at all times is

The rule of consistency

The rule of consistency is simple: However you choose to use the ideas in this book, they can only work in your home, with your child or children, if you use them the same way every day and at every mealtime. I do not mean that if I suggest that family meals should be together that you *have* to have all meals together. But that if you do have, say, one meal per day together, that everyone joins in, every day.

Decide what you are going to do and what your rules will be and then stick to them.

Say, for example, that you have agreed a family rule that anyone who has not eaten their main course doesn't have any pudding. If you waver or give in even once – for instance, if the pudding is a special cake that you have made for Sunday lunch and you decide that it is not fair if someone misses out on it - you will put the idea in the heads of your offspring that they can get away with not doing as you have said. The next mealtime, they will almost certainly nag, pester and manipulate you if you try to reassert yourself and stick to the rule that you yourself broke the day before!

The most important thing you can do to achieve consistently is to positively *reinforce* and *reward* the behaviours that you want and *ignore* the behaviours you do not want. This is the way that many children learn what is acceptable and not acceptable in their own homes and out in the rest of society. It is what most child experts suggest will be effective in making children well-adjusted and happy in their own choices as they grow up. Many examples are given in the next pages.

Remember: be consistent – reward the behaviours you want – ignore the behaviours you do not want.

Some Ground Rules

Rule 1: get into a routine

It is a good idea to get into some routine with regards when and how meals are eaten as early as possible. One reason for doing this is that when children go to nursery, pre-school and school, they will be expected to sit and eat meals with other children. If you want your child to start eating with you as early as possible, getting him or her to have regular large meals will develop the concept of mealtimes (rather than other times) being when food is eaten.

Adults who do not have a good routine around eating are unable to monitor either what they eat or their calorie intake. If you do not establish some sort of structure for your children's mealtimes, you won't be able to keep a real eye on what they are eating and you could easily fall into the trap of not knowing whether your child is hungry or just trying to be in control.

When my children first started eating proper food, we had the following sort of routine:

Between 7am and 8am	Breakfast
Between 10am and 11am	Drink and snack
Around 1pm	Lunch
Between 3pm and 3.30pm	Drink and snack
Between 5.30pm and 6.30pm	Tea

After tea it was bath, teeth, book and bed by around 7pm.

Clearly, we did not always stick rigidly to these times and you need to apply some reason to the routine that you choose. If you are out shopping and it gets to 11am and you have not managed to stop and give your toddler a drink and his or her usual banana, it is not going to matter. In our house, when the children were very little, bedtime determined the time of breakfast. If they woke at their usual time (between 5.30 and 6.30 am) and breakfast was later than about 8am, both of them would start to be really hungry and often a fight would break out (thus delaying breakfast by even more.) But if they had been somewhere with us and had a late dinner, they might sleep later in the morning and breakfast would be later, too. And although the nursery had lunch at 11.30am, this was replaced by a later morning snack if the children were at home, which kept them going until our "proper" lunchtime.

Children do like routines and repetition. Much more than adults do. Think about how many times they want to watch their favourite DVD – I'm convinced I can recite the script of "Bambi!" That is another reason why establishing some fairly fixed mealtimes is a good idea. They like to know what comes next in their day and that tea will be at teatime.

Rule 2: give your child as many different things to eat as you can

There is a relatively small period of time during which your child's eating preferences are established. Sometimes this is referred to as a "window of opportunity". Between six months and about a year old, if a baby has a broad range of tastes and textures to enjoy, then they are more likely to continue to be happy to eat lots of different foods. If their choice during this period is limited to pureed apple, mashed potato and children's yoghurts, their taste for other foods may be stifled.

My alternative wording of this rule is "encourage the gourmand." This is important right through the early years of childhood and onwards. What you want is a little person who will appreciate and enjoy all food. So if you can get everyone in the family eating lots of different, new foods and talking about them, this is going to be something that is exciting for the children. They are going to want to explore new food tastes and textures and will not be intimidated by unfamiliar dishes. Think about a child's social development. As they come into contact with your friends and their peers, they are probably going to attend a series of events which revolve around food – birthday parties and weddings, for example. Although fun, such occasions can also be fairly stressful for parents and child alike. Do you want your child to be anxious that he or she will not like the food at a friend's house, their school or the nursery picnic? Or do you want to equip them with enough experience and knowledge of all sorts of food so that this is at least one area of a new event that neither they or you will need to worry about?

Even before a baby is born they have been influenced in what they will choose to eat by what their mother ate. Research with pregnant women who ate various foods, including garlic, anise and carrot juice, found that their children were more likely to eat these foods than those with mothers who had avoided them.[xxi] This also supports the principle that it is familiarity with a wide range of foods, as early as possible, that will encourage babies and children to achieve enjoyment of food generally.

I found weaning quite stressful – worrying about what to feed my baby with right at the beginning and how much she should have and when. If you are unsure what to start with, buy a book to help you. There are some fantastic titles on the shelves, covering weaning and older childrens' diets and many of them provide full menu plans from week one onwards.[xxii] They often start off with fruit and vegetable purees, with or without milk and baby rice mixed in. From the age at which your baby can eat a wider range of foods, such as meat, eggs, fish and wheat, they progress to a full range of meal options, which can be made in advance and frozen if you need to save time.

My main criticism of these books is that they start you, the food-preparer and cook, off on the journey of making separate meals for the children. There is more about this in chapter 5, as it can become quite a problem for some families. At first, it may seem the most sensible option - your nine-month old baby may not be as ecstatic as you are at the prospect of vindaloo curry for dinner. However, the principle of introducing the broadest variety possible must, surely, include the things that we all eat, all of the time. In other words, maybe you *should* try them on curry at nine months - albeit one with limited hot spice included. My children did eat very mild curries from about the age of one year. Although we did once have a guilt-ridden incident with thai fish cakes and a chilli garnish during a pub lunch: My daughter, who was not yet two, thought the chilli was red pepper.

You will also find that many of the meals that are suggested in these children's recipe books are simply "babyfied" versions of the real thing. The book that I used when my daughter started to eat solid foods included recipes for boeuf bourguignon (yes, really), fish chowder and vegetable soup. I could have made them using a standard cookery book and saved the cover price. So my suggestion is that, as early as you feel able, you ask yourself "is it really necessary to make a pasta dish just for the baby, when I am going to be cooking a pasta meal for myself/ourselves, anyway?" There is nothing wrong with mashed-up lasagne, after all.

Rule 3: don't start them off on the junk

There is a clear exception to the previous rule: it refers, of course to all kinds of "junk" food. Thinking on this varies. Some people don't let their children eat any sweet things before the age of two. Others feel that a little sweet food will do no harm at any age. What I have noticed is how many foods targeted at babies and young children are really packed with sugars and salts. The two that readily spring to mind are children's yoghurts or fromage frais and breakfast cereals.

My daughter likes a little chocolate. But she usually can't manage a whole piece of cake. She often tells me that something is too sweet for her. You could put this down to genetics or you could say that these preferences are because she wasn't given any sweet foods until she was about eighteen months old. Nevertheless, given the choice, she would rather have a piece of fruit than a piece of cake. That makes it a lot easier for us to make sure she eats her five fruit and vegetable portions every day with no hint of complaint.

My son loves potatoes, bread and other starchy foods, although when presented with a plate of food, he will often eat the vegetables first, followed by the meat and then the potatoes. He also enjoys sweet things more than his sister. Again, this could be genetic. But when he was a baby he was often given cake and bits of chocolate by both us and his extended family. If my daughter was having a cake, it didn't seem fair to deny it to her younger brother. So I believe he has built up more of a "taste" for sweet, starchy foods. Because of the way we eat as a family, I am not bothered about this. But I would be if he preferred these foods and took every opportunity to demand them, rather than eating the healthier options we provide.

The point is that I think that children are "programmed" to like starchy, sweet foods and there is some research evidence to support this. One explanation is that these foods supply energy and, in a situation where food is scarce, this preference improves the chances of survival. Going back to our cave-living forbears, this seems a sensible approach. Children need relatively more energy-giving foods than adults do. But if the exposure to these foods is balanced with even more exposure to healthier foods – fresh fruit and vegetables, home-cooked meals and wholemeal variations of food – then there is no reason why your child should ever develop a craving or physical dependence upon them.

From a nutritional perspective, you should be aware that neither your body, nor your children's bodies require sugar and fatty foods to stay healthy. Sugar and other "poor" foods will simply take the place of those things which are better for us and can therefore limit the ability of our bodies to obtain the optimum range of nutrients. If you expose your child to sugary sweets and chocolate, but not to, say, the natural sweetness of a ripe pineapple or chewy date, you are restricting the other aspects of experiencing food – texture, smell and so on. I love making cakes for my children. The look on their faces when they take a bite gives me a huge amount of pleasure. But I am also conscious of the fact that I get a warm feeling from that which is equally if not more rewarding to me than the feeling they get from eating the cake. I only make cakes occasionally and puddings, snacks and sweets are probably less than twice-weekly events for the family. My friend, who is a clinical nutritionist once said to me "Examine your conscience when you bake a cake: are you doing it for them or for yourself?"

Think carefully and check the nutritional content of the food you buy, especially the amount of sugar, starch and other carbohydrate-based ingredients. If sugar, glucose syrup or similar is the second ingredient on the list, that means there is lots of it in there. If you want to read the nutritional information on the packet, anything that says it has more than 10g or sugar per 100g of product is not a high-quality food option for your family. Try to think about the overall balance of foods you offer and minimise the amount of rubbish your child eats.

Rule 4: discard your pre-conceptions and prejudices about what a child should eat

We understand that a baby is more likely to want a varied diet as they get older if they are given lots of different things before the age of one. But how do parents know what foods are suitable or not suitable for their baby? One thing that I have observed is how parents make judgements about what their children should eat and that these do not appear to be based on anything other than their own personal belief. In other words, there is no rationale to the decision – it is based upon some kind of pre-conceived idea about "what children eat."

We went to the house of a friend for pre-Christmas nibbles. One of the things on offer was smoked salmon and cream cheese "pinwheels". Our children ate these among the other things on offer. However, the parents whose house we were in didn't let their little girl eat any of the smoked salmon. I asked why and they simply said that they didn't think it was a "good idea."

I think that this is not about what is suitable. Most foods are perfectly safe and acceptable to feed to a small child. We have already covered the issue of food intolerance and allergies – they really are less of a problem than many of us think. I believe there is a self-generated issue about what our children actually should be given to eat. A kind of framework, or set of boxes, into which types of food are mentally placed. So, there would be the box for "feed from age six months" – that will be the pureed vegetables and fruit, then, and one for "able to eat from five years" – I think that applies to boiled sweets, whole nuts and uncooked eggs, such as in fresh mayonnaise.

But it is deeper than that. There are some parents who seem to be worried that their children are eating the wrong things all the time. And I am not talking about sweets. I am talking about everyday foods. Lots of people appear to worry about whether their children will get an upset tummy from eating too much fruit. Others are apparently concerned about spicy food, bitter or sharp-tasting food, slimy foods. Where exactly is it written down that a child will not like grapefruit? Or curry? What about aubergines or mackerel? It may be that you do not like these things, but shouldn't you assume that a baby or small child, tasting something for the first time, will be excited by that new smell, taste and texture? Once you start to apply your mental "rules" about what the little one will eat, you are restricting the range of experiences of food for that child. Please forgive me for saying this, but your rules are almost certainly based on hearsay, personal preferences and family history – and probably have very little to do with healthy eating and the science of nutrition.

Here is another story. We went to a restaurant with a family who are friends. Our children and their children are about the same age. It was a pizza restaurant - not anything exotic. The parents of the other children analysed the menu in detail. And within the hearing of their children they were saying:

Dad: "How about this pasta with tomato sauce?"
Mum: "Well, she's a bit funny about tomatoes."
Dad: "What about the lasagne?"
Mum: "She hasn't had it before -I don't think she'll eat it."
Dad: "Shall we give her a pizza?"
Mum: "It might be a bit tough for her."
Dad: "Well, we could get her some dough-balls, or something."
Mum: "Yes, that'll be OK."

Their beliefs and self-imposed construct of "what my child would like to eat," were over-laying the child's idea about what she should eat. Her perception of food was being coloured by these exchanges in her early life. She was not yet two years old, but before she had opened her mouth, she was being given a series of fairly negative messages about the food that was available in the restaurant. If she *had* been given the lasagne to eat, do you think she would have eaten it, after her mother had said she probably wouldn't? Not surprisingly, we did notice that these otherwise lovely children had a limited range of food that they liked to eat and as they have grown older this has remained the case.

If you can get rid of all those ideas in *your* head about what your little ones will enjoy, you can become a true advocate for a broad range of food and drink for all the family.

Rule 5: say the right things

Your role as a parent is to provide as many exciting opportunities as possible for your children to eat lots of different foods. Part of that role also includes being consistently positive and encouraging about eating new foods. You influence so much of what your children do unconsciously – through what you say and how you behave. For example, how should you speak about food in front of younger members of the family? Most people are not even aware that the words that come from their mouths can have a huge influence on how their children think of the food in front of them. Look at the list that follows and think about whether you have said anything from the right hand side of the table recently. Ask yourself how this makes the food seem to your two, three or five-year old.

Do say	Don't say
Look, Ben, something new today	I am not sure you have had this before
You're going to like this	I don't know if you'll like this
Yes, go on, try it	I think you'd better not have that
Are you going to try that? Daddy (Or Mummy) will have some, too	You're a bit young for that
Nothing at all – just let them get on with it	It looks a bit odd/yucky/off, doesn't it?
Mmm, it is (or looks) really juicy/tasty/yummy - anything which you think is a positive attribute of the food	Mummy (or Daddy) doesn't really like that, but you might

When you give your child something different to eat it should not be a major event or a "big thing". You want your baby or toddler to understand that eating new foods is a normal part of everyday life. Your voice, what you say and how you look should convey to the little one that it is interesting and good to eat new things. There should be no doubt in your mind that your child will like what he or she is about to eat. If there *is* any doubt, it will almost certainly show in your face. This will be as good as saying to your son or daughter, "I don't know if you'll like this," or something similar. Be careful with your body-language.

Don't forget that you are the role model and you have to be positive. An important aspect of being positive relates to what foods you will eat yourself. Obviously, if there are many things you do not like, you are already potentially restricting the range of meals you child will eat and enjoy. If you find it a challenge to try out new foods yourself, then it will be harder for you to convey the right message to your children and I think this can be a big issue. So from now on you need to say firmly to yourself "I enjoy trying new foods and usually like them" – rather than "I am worried that I won't like this food."

Rule 6: reward the behaviour you want and ignore the behaviour you do not want

Your child knows when it has done the right thing, because you smile and say "Good girl/boy" and you might even get quite excited about it. You can use the same positive, rewarding behaviours when your child eats or drinks something for the first time. You need to reinforce what you want to see - your children eating what they have on their plates - and basically ignore what you do not want to happen, which is your children refusing food, spitting it out, or other types of behaviour which you want to stop. If you are consistent in what you say and in what you do, you are providing a set of positive experiences related to eating food. Even the smallest babies will pick these cues up and start to associate mealtimes with smiles, happy faces and a general sense of well-being.

Here is a summary of the ground rules I have set out above:
1. Get into a routine
2. Give your child as many different things to eat as you can
3. Don't start them off on the junk
4. Discard your pre-conceptions and prejudices about what a child should eat
5. Say the right things
6. Reward the behaviour you want and ignore the behaviour you do not want.

How to Make Sure They Eat What You Give Them

Rule 7: if food is refused, offer it again at a later time and keep on doing it

This is an important rule because you may already have noticed that little babies and toddlers sometimes pull a face when you give them something new to try. My children did that, too. Does this mean that she or he doesn't like what they have been given? I don't know. Sometimes a baby or toddler will actually *shudder* when they eat something. The other behaviour is refusal of a food – mouth clamped shut and/or head turned - often followed by the little one pushing the dish or bowl away. This is both worrying and quite off-putting. Especially when you have just spent an hour making carrot, apple and parsnip mash for their lunch and there are another ten tiny portions sitting on the kitchen table ready to pop into the freezer! Ask yourself a couple of questions: "Am I going to assume that my baby doesn't like carrots, apple and parsnips and not give them to him or her any more?" and "What am I going to do the next time my child pulls a face or pushes the bowl away?" What could happen is that your child starts to make faces or push food away because he or she gets a reaction from you – you look worried or anxious, or try and jolly them into eating some more, or sing to them while they are eating. Bear in mind that babies and toddlers crave attention of any kind – an interesting reaction is a reward which is almost as good as a cuddle or kiss.

Now think about what happens if you decide to not give your child that particular food again. You have "deleted" something from your list of foods that he or she likes. Next time, you delete something else, then again and again. So, you are funnelling down into an ever-more limited group of foods that the little one will eat. If you do this now, how easy will it be to encourage them back into eating these foods as they get older? Especially once they can negotiate and argue with you.

When my daughter was very little I gave her a mixture of mashed-up pasta, cauliflower and cheese to eat, She spat the first mouthful out and then every other one. When I tried her on pasta again, she did the same thing. But in my mind I could see years ahead of me in which I would cook pasta for the rest of the family (maybe two or three times a week) and something else for my daughter. I decided to keep giving her pasta.

I was not being mean to her. I knew that research shows that repeated experience of a food – up to ten times - leads to acceptance. For a very young child, there is no reason for them to dislike *any* food. The expression on their face (and the shuddering!) is probably because they have never yet had that exact combination of smell, taste and texture. Like anyone, they may need to try it a few more times before they get used to it. My advice is in two stages.

First, don't respond to the negative behaviour. Remember, we are ignoring behaviours we do not want to be repeated. If your little boy or girl doesn't eat the food after several spoonfuls have been attempted, quietly clear it away and get on with the next thing you had planned for your day. You can tell him or her what you are doing – "I am going to clear your lunch away, now, because you don't seem to want it. Perhaps you will be hungry later at teatime". This is not producing any interesting response from you, as far as your baby or toddler is concerned.

Second, put the little pots in the freezer and get one out every couple of days for a meal. You will be able to get your child to keep trying the food because he or she is unlikely to realise that the meal offered on Tuesday is the same as the meal that was not eaten on Friday. Whatever you do, don't say "we tried this last week, but you didn't want it, so let's try it again". Another tactic is to vary the "mix" on the plate. For example, you might feed your baby the carrot, apple and parsnip alongside some plain carrot. When I used to do this, I was convinced that my baby was "mulling over" the different tastes on the plate. Even if you have to keep offering the same meal a few times, your baby will eat it at some point. And then you will have the confidence to offer that food again and to be consistent next time something is refused. Don't give in when a face is pulled or the food pot pushed away.

Remember also to apply rule number six. Provide plenty of encouragement and reward in the way of smiles and positive feedback when your child does eat the food that he or she may have previously rejected.

(By-the-way, my daughter loves pasta).

Rule 8: never offer an alternative

Should you give your baby something else to try when he has refused to eat what you first offered? I don't think so and here is why.

Weaning gives you the first chance to set the rules about eating, without there being the likelihood that your child is left feeling hungry. The reason is because, while you are gradually encouraging the consumption of solid food, the main nutrients of your baby's diet are still provided by the milk she or he drinks. If baby decides not to eat a meal, it really doesn't matter.

We went to visit some friends and stayed the night at their house. Their little girl was less than two years old. Our friends had only just moved in and the dining table was not big enough for all of us to eat round it, so we gave the children their food first and then ate ourselves afterwards. At breakfast time, the little girl didn't eat anything she was offered - wheat cereal and some fruit juice. When we sat down to eat *our* breakfast, she sidled up to her mother and asked for some of her toast - and was given it! "Never mind if you don't eat your meal, you can just come back and ask me later and I will find you something else that you feel like eating. Probably from my own plate". At the time, I was amazed, because this was a clever, generally sensible person. And she had just done something I would never have considered: when the food that was offered was refused, she provided an alternative.

What your child will eat in the longer term is going to be decided by how you behave and the rules you set. If a baby or toddler pulls a face and refuses any more of the food you have prepared, you could say "oh dear, don't you like that? I'll find you something else", then go to the fridge and get out something which you know your baby definitely will eat. The reason you do this is because you do not want him or her to be hungry. The lesson for the mealtime will have been "if I don't want something, I pull a face and don't eat it and Mummy/Daddy will get me something I like". You are effectively rewarding your child for not eating the food that you gave him or her. In this way, it will only take a few weeks and months for your child to be the dictator of much of what he or she eats.

On the other hand, you could say, "oh, not hungry? Never mind, you can try it again tomorrow" and clear the dishes. The lesson for that mealtime being "If I don't eat my food, Daddy/Mummy assumes I am not hungry and that is the end of the meal". Furthermore, when tomorrow comes around, if the food is presented again and the same thing happens, you are already setting the ground-rule that nothing else is offered but the food available for that mealtime, so it is up to baby to decide whether they eat or not. I know that it took very few mealtimes for both of our children to start to understand that the food that they were given was what they were supposed to eat and that if they did not eat it, there was no other option available. You *have* to be consistent with applying this approach. Tiny children learn very quickly. If you are consistent one, two or three times, you will probably never have this issue arise again – or, at least, not until your children are older and you can discuss with them directly that there is no alternative to the food on offer.

This may feel like a very tough thing to do, but ask yourself: "Do I want my child to argue about food at every meal or would I like him or her just to eat what I give them, unconditionally?" Remember that only a child who is really not that hungry will be able to consistently refuse food for mealtime after mealtime. The reason our children can do this is because they are fed more than they actually need to eat. A baby or toddler who is still drinking milk as a large proportion of their daily nutritional intake may never be really hungry. Remember also that children learn very quickly and are actually comfortable with rules, routines and frameworks in which everyone is treated the same. Finally, remember that it is normal for children to eat a lot for one mealtime or on one particular day and then to eat practically nothing at another mealtime or on another day. Any health visitor or GP will tell you that no harm will come to a healthy child just because he or she has missed one or even two meals.

It is *really important* that you *do not give in*. This is why. As babies we basically all learn through reward. If we get something right, we get some kind of positive outcome. If we eat our food, for example, someone smiles at us. If we are ignored for what we are doing, we are not being rewarded, so we stop doing whatever it is. Imagine a scenario where you have just tried to give your little one some mashed potato and beans for lunch and s/he has refused to eat it, despite a good few tries on your part. "Ok", you say, "we'll leave it for now and maybe you will eat more at teatime". So far, so good. But now your baby starts crying. They cry and cry and are obviously quite agitated. They keep on crying and you are getting more and more stressed. At last, you give in and get one of the nice baby yoghurts out of the fridge. What have you just rewarded your child for? Crying. If you do this, your child will quickly make a connection between crying and getting the food that he or she likes. Next time, you might feel more determined and leave it longer before you give in. You will be training your child to cry for longer to get what he or she wants! If you stick to your resolve and refuse to give in right from the start, you will never start this cycle off.

I know a little boy who can pick and choose his food, because his Mum gives in to him when he says he is hungry: although he doesn't eat much at mealtimes, he somehow manages to get a lot of snack food down. He just never eats his main meals. I cannot imagine how frustrating that must be for his mother, but she has indirectly caused the situation to occur because she doesn't have the confidence to choose to make him go hungry a couple of times. And she has not set out and stuck to clear rules for both herself and him to follow.

Again, I know this is a hard thing to do, but *be firm* and stick to what you have decided to do. Do not give in. Do not feel guilty. Think about the long term: whatever you feel now, it will be nothing compared to years of worrying about whether your children are eating enough of the right things to keep them healthy now and in the future.

Rule 9: adapt snack arrangements to maintain an appetite for proper meals

When you apply rule number eight, you might also need to think about intervals between meals. Many children I know – including my own – are fed up to five times every day. This is because of the habit of offering snacks in between main meals. Between breakfast and lunch there is the mid-morning snack and between lunch and dinner (or tea-time) is the mid-afternoon snack. My children's nursery seemed to offer food every couple of hours, although I suspect this was just to give the carers a break and some time to tidy up!

The problem with snacks is that a child can feel full before a meal – rather than being hungry and ready to eat. Snacks are often high in calories. Even a small banana will fill a child up if it is eaten only an hour and a half before a meal. This opens the door wide to selective refusal of food that is deemed too crunchy, mushy, green or otherwise unpleasant to eat. It makes it much easier to tell Daddy or Mummy "I don't like that" if you're not actually hungry. Now, if it was a banana and a biscuit, like I had an hour and a half ago, I might give it a go......

If my children didn't eat any of their lunch, I always made it very clear that there would be nothing else until tea-time. If your little girl or boy is consistently refusing some or all items of food within their main meal, while happily eating snacks, then it is likely that the snack food is a substitute for the main meal. By its very nature, snack food is less nourishing and often less healthy than most main meals. You therefore need to decide which of the following to do:

a) Stop giving snacks (at least until main meals are "on the menu" again)
b) Minimise snacks – for example, only offer a single piece of fruit (small apple or pear, satsuma or similar) as a snack, so that your child is less likely to find it substantial enough to substitute for larger meals
c) Only give a snack if the previous main meal was eaten.

Rule 10: give your child a portion of food that you can reasonably expect them to eat

The most sensible way to maximise the likelihood that everything will be eaten is to start off with really small portions. For the very youngest child, who is still reliant on milk for most of their nutritional needs, even tiny amounts of food that are eaten should be rewarded with big smiles.

Take the path of least resistance: if you start with a small portion of food on the plate, the chances are that all of it will get eaten. And that means that you can provide immediate, positive feedback – in the form of smiles, verbal cues, such as "good girl, well done, you ate it all!" and in the option of offering more of what your child wants to eat. This is much easier for you than trying to force an unwilling baby or toddler to eat what may seem to them like a mountain of a meal – even if it is only three tablespoons of food. To him or her that could look like loads and loads of fish pie and vegetables – and it comes with a massive bottle or cup of really filling milk! No wonder, then, if what is consumed turns out to be the stuff they know they like – the mashed potato topping – and not the small pile of cabbage that came with it.

You can start each meal by giving your child just a teaspoon of each separate element on their plate. This is what I call a "mini meal" and it can be a useful approach for older children, too. A mini meal might be a teaspoon of fish pie, a teaspoon of sweetcorn and a teaspoon of cabbage. Even for an adult, a full teaspoon is enough for them a get a proper taste and feel of that food, so that they become familiar with it. You don't need them to eat a lot of something in one meal for your little girl or boy to go from not being sure whether they like a food to being sure that they *do* like it. It is not a problem if they need to try that type of food, say, six times at six different meals, for them to build the necessary experience to learn to enjoy its uniqueness.

Once the mini meal has been eaten, you can put some more of everything on the plate. It might be two teaspoonfuls this time, to make things go faster. Once you have gained some confidence that your child or children will eat what you give them at every mealtime, you can gradually increase the size of the mini meal, giving them a larger portion at the start of the meal – rather than adding small amounts to an empty plate every few minutes. You should feel a real sense of satisfaction that you have cooked a meal, put it in front of them and watched it being eaten. However, be aware of any bad habits that may come creeping back. For instance, you may start to make an allowance that not everything on their plates is eaten once you are giving them a proper meal in one go. But make sure that it is not consistently the vegetables that are being pushed to one side, or the other things that you suspect your toddler prefers to avoid. If this starts to happen, switch back to the mini meal system straight away. If, over a period of time, main courses are never being finished, then review the amount you are putting on the plate and act accordingly.

Rule 11: you must always try all the food on your plate

The wording of this rule is intentional – it includes you and all of the other adults in your family, too.

Once they reached the age of about two or three and started to take notice of what other little girls and boys said, my own children would occasionally tell me they didn't like a particular food on their plate.

We have a clear set of rules regarding how we talk about food and how we treat food and there is more about this later in the book. One rule is that we always try things. Even Daddy, who – as I have explained – struggles with many foods, will try things properly and make sure the children know that he has done so. The purpose of getting someone to try something is threefold:

First, as adults, we know that the food on our plate will not harm us or our children. But evolution has hard-wired in a sense of doubt in the baby or toddler's mind. You therefore have to be the advocate of that particular food item – whether it is some mashed swede, a piece of bacon or a funny-coloured pink and orange ice-cream (hopefully not, though). If you encourage your child to try everything, they will quickly learn that there are no foods that they need to be frightened of.

Second, we already know that exposure to a wide variety of food is a good thing. So making sure that as many things are tried as possible is the logical next step of this process.

Finally, I think that we should be teaching children that trying foods and making an effort to enjoy them is part of respecting food. I have written more about this in relation to older children, too. But, in essence, babies and toddlers should be expected to eat what they are given – in the old-fashioned sense of that phrase "Well, when we were children, we were just expected to eat what was on our plates". I have yet to find anyone who fundamentally disagrees with my opinion in this area.

You may find it useful, if your child says they do not like something, to talk to him or her about whether there is a reason that they don't like it. I find that our children sometimes say they don't like something. Or they leave one component of their meal for a long time on their plate and I might be watching them, thinking "oh-oh, looks like they might leave that". But when they try the food, they actually either like it or don't mind eating it, so they'll eat the rest of the portion. Sometimes, however, things are slimy or mushy or have some other feature that a child finds difficult to deal with. You might choose to tell your little one that foods have all sorts of tastes and textures – that is partly what is interesting about eating - and you are trying to help them get used to as many as possible, so that they will like lots of things when they grow up. It is fine to talk through the various merits and issues around food (including how you may have cooked it!) if this will help a child to carry on trying everything.

Trying a food means having a proper mouthful. A teaspoonful will do – it is just enough for you to be able to properly taste and feel the food in your mouth. There is no point in plonking a large dollop of food down and refusing to let your child leave the table until he or she has eaten it. As long as the little one has put the spoonful in, chewed it and swallowed it, then you should be satisfied that he or she has made a good effort to try the food.

The more different things your family eats, the more confident all of you will feel about new things and about eating in unfamiliar situations. A big part of how happy and secure your children will feel about going out to see friends, to make school trips, to being invited out to restaurants will be how used they are to trying and then eating anything they are given.

At my daughter's fourth birthday party we gave the children cream cheese sandwiches cut into teddy bear shapes, cherry tomatoes, cucumber, carrot and pepper sticks with hummus, a few crisps and cheesy biscuits, olives, fruit salad and an "owl and the pussy cat" birthday cake! Seven of the eight children who were there really enjoyed their meal. But one little girl just said "I don't like that" to almost everything on the table. In the end, she ate some crisps and a piece of birthday cake. Her grandmother was with her and said "try this", "try this". But it was obvious that the child wasn't used to trying anything and wasn't about to start now. You would think this type of behaviour would be catching, wouldn't you? The sad truth is that this one little girl was really left out, because none of the other children understood what was going on: they just ignored her and carried on eating – everything.

A few months later we met this little girl again, with her family, at a local country house estate. We all went to have lunch in the courtyard café. Our children had an egg salad with a jacket potato followed by some fruit. The little girl and her brother ate white bread ham sandwiches and a bag of crisps. We offered them some cucumber sticks, but they weren't interested. At one point their mother said – almost proudly – "she only eats peas and carrots". I thought this was a bit sad and simply a reflection of how they had allowed their youngsters to grow up without getting them to even try anything.

The rules I have covered in this section are:

7. If food is refused, offer it again at a later time and keep on doing it
8. Never offer an alternative
9. Adapt snack arrangements to maintain an appetite for proper meals
10. Give your child a portion of food that you can reasonably expect them to eat
11. You must always try all the food on your plate.

Supporting Strategies

Rule 12: make it clear what happens if they eat the food and what happens if they don't – and stick to it

Even very young children soon learn and understand the consequences of their own actions or decision. You can use something which can be expressed as "if….then….but" to set the expectation of your child about what the consequences of their decisions will be. This process places your child in the driving seat, because it allows them to choose for themselves: they can either eat what you are offering them, or they can decide not to eat it. If they eat the food, they will be rewarded, but if they don't they will not.

My sister's little girl is a sweet thing with a strong will, who developed a clear dislike of fruit. This caused huge anxiety to her Mum and Dad, who, like many people, see fruit snacks as a good way of achieving the five-a-day goal with their children. Despite all their best efforts, they could really only get her to eat bananas, and there is a limit to the number of bananas you want a child to eat in a day (they are very filling, after all). Once, the little girl came to stay with Grandma and her two cousins for a holiday. She was about eighteen months old and just a couple of months younger than her next oldest cousin. For breakfast every day, the children were given a small bowl of fruit, such as apple and pear and this was followed by some toast with whatever they would like on top. On the first morning, the little one didn't want her small portion of fruit. She kept saying "Toast.".So we said to her "Yes, when you have had some fruit." But she didn't want her fruit - she wanted some toast. We carried on telling her that she *could* have toast, as long as she ate some fruit, but this didn't work, so we then explained that we were about to clear away the breakfast things. I think that right up until the last minute, she thought we would give in and let her eat the toast alone.

The outcome of that meal was that she didn't have any breakfast. She was very cross and cried a lot and screamed for a bit, but she still didn't have any breakfast. Next day for breakfast she ate her fruit and her toast.

The "if....then....but" approach sets some clear rules about what is expected of your child at mealtimes. It works even on really young children from about eighteen months old, because, as I have said, they do understand the results and consequences of their own decisions at a very early age. Here is an example of how you might set the expectation of the consequences of a child's choice:

Dad: "Tom, if you eat that plateful, you can have seconds of anything that you want."
Tom: "Can I have some more mashed potatoes?"
Dad: "Please.....yes you can have more mashed potatoes if you eat all of that."
Tom: "I like mashed potatoes best."
Dad: "Yes, I know. Eat it up."
Tom: "What are these green things?"
Dad: "They're called mange-tout. I really like them."
Tom: "I don't like it."
Dad: "Well, that's OK, but if you don't eat it all, you won't be able to have any more of the mashed potato, so could you eat it, please."

Dad is making it clear that there is a reward for eating the food on the plate – including the mange-tout. He is being encouraging without making too much fuss. He is also being assertive about what he wants to happen – he wants everything to be eaten.

Here is another example:
Lily: "Mum, I don't like cabbage."
Mum: "Well, you have had it before and it tastes the same every time."

Lily: "Yes, but I don't like it."

Mum: "Lily, I am not interested in whether you like it or not, because you have started saying this about all sorts of nice foods. You know the rule: you need to try everything on your plate. If you eat the cabbage, you can watch that new DVD this afternoon, but if you do not you will have to find something else to do instead."

Lily: "But I don't want it."

Mum: "Lily, that is fine. I would like you to try the cabbage, please. If you do eat a good mouthful, while I am watching, you can put the DVD on. Otherwise, the meal is over and you will need to find something else to do."

Lily: "I don't want it."

Mum: "I am not discussing it further. I have explained the situation to you - please will you eat some of the cabbage."

The message you should be giving must be consistent and you may find yourself repeating it over and over, as in the example. "Please will you eat what I have given you (or, at least, try it)." Very young children should not be negotiating with you, so be firm and just stick to the original statement: if you eat the food, then you can have the reward. If you do not eat the food, that is not a problem for me (you are ignoring the behaviour you do not want), but you need to be aware that there is no reward for you.

There is no need at all to give your child more food as a reward for eating their meal. In fact, it is generally agreed that it is not a great idea to use foods as rewards – especially things like puddings, sweets and cakes. These, after all, should be occasional foods – not everyday parts of our children's diets. My children were always very keen to earn stickers. They liked the option to have an extra book read to them at bedtime, or to go to the park after lunch. Your children may want to see a DVD, go swimming, have a magazine to read or listen to their favourite music CD. Rather than thinking about this as an exercise in eating food, try to view it within the framework of "good behaviour" and choose your rewards accordingly.

At a meal at home, my little boy knew that there was some cake which was available for pudding. He just kept asking for the cake and ignored what was on his plate. Over and over again, I said, "Yes, you can have some cake, when you have eaten your food, but if you don't eat what is on your plate, you won't be able to have any cake", but still nothing was eaten. I felt terrible as he was carried upstairs for his bath crying and screaming and demanding cake, while his sister tucked in to hers with a huge smile on her face. But I had to be consistent and I had to be clear: you do not get rewarded for not eating your food. It can be very tough, but if you are consistent and firm and don't give in, your life and the life of your child will be easier from an early age and this will carry on into the rest of their childhood.

Some people avoid this issue by never mentioning that there is cake or pudding to come before the first course has been eaten. I think that this does work, to some extent, but wouldn't it be easier if you could give everyone their main course and they would eat it, regardless of whether they were expecting a pudding, or not?

What if all of the meal before bedtime is refused?

It is one thing being tough about what your child has refused to eat at lunchtime, when you know there is another opportunity for filling up later on in the day. It is quite a different matter when the meal that is completely refused is the last one of the day and your child will have to get through to breakfast on an empty stomach. I think this is a particular dilemma for parents of children up to about age three. Obviously, you don't want your child to be really hungry when they wake up – or, worse, to wake up in the night because they really need something to eat.

This is a real pitfall for the parent or carer seeking to be consistent about rules applied to mealtimes. However, try to assess (if you know) what your child has eaten during the afternoon. You may realise that actually he or she has had quite a lot to eat and can probably manage to go through the night without another meal. A friend whose child was at the same nursery as my son and daughter told me that she never bothered to give him a meal after she picked him up in the afternoon. That meant that the little boy had no meal between 3.30 or 4.00pm and breakfast the next day. At the time, I was surprised, but it never seemed to cause any problems. Often, my children were not hungry after nursery, because they had just eaten all day and there was always plenty of food in their tummies. If they didn't eat a lot of their tea I would worry about whether they would be hungry and wake up in the night. But I don't remember that they ever did.

If you really cannot bear to put your child to bed after they have refused to eat any of their last meal of the day, then I suggest you offer only something very light to eat. Maybe a piece of fruit, such as a small apple, or a plain cracker – very boring, yet sustaining if required – and a drink of water. Another option is a glass of milk. Do not forget that your toddler has made a choice not to eat his or her meal: you offered good food and he or she decided not to eat it. Remind yourself that this can only happen when a child is basically not hungry. Don't give in and offer the little one a yoghurt or a banana, or a piece of toast and marmite. A small piece of fruit or a cracker will be enough.

Rule 13: don't make a fuss

Over and over again, media articles and books about children and food say "don't make a fuss" if meals are not eaten. I agree with this principle, but I think that parents have misinterpreted it to mean "don't do anything and carry on as if nothing has happened". This never worked for me. If I cook a main meal which is not eaten, I am not going to carry on as if nothing had happened and produce a lovely pudding for everyone to eat instead. This is contradictory to rule number eight which says not to offer an alternative. "Don't you want your lasagne? Never mind, have some trifle, instead".

My interpretation of "don't make a fuss" is to make clear what the options are; offer them and then act upon the decision made. When I say, "don't make a fuss", then, I mean just get on with it. I have already covered why nothing else should be offered to a baby or toddler who has refused a meal or who won't even taste their carrots. The actions that go with this decision are: state what you are doing and do it. Move on to the next thing. Here is an example of what I mean:

Mum: "Look, you're having the same as me today"
Francis: "Blargh, blug, dub"
Mum: "It's lovely, try it again"
Francis: "Splurt, splat, ugh"
Mum: "Do you want some more?"
Francis: "Nah!"
Mum: "Ok, but there isn't anything else to eat. Are you sure?"
Francis: "Nah!"
Mum: "Alright. Let's clear away and we'll go and find a book to read".

So in this case "not making a fuss" means not taking any notice of the behaviour that you really don't want to see again - i.e. refusing the food. If you combine this with the positive reinforcement that you give if the little one eats what they are given, you will be well on the road to making it "normal" for them to eat everything that they are given.

The other type of fuss-making, which you quite often see with very little children is "Daddy is an aeroplane". It is tempting, isn't it? If Baby isn't eating very well or simply refusing to eat, Daddy gets some food on the spoon and pretends that it is a train going into a tunnel or an aeroplane coming in to land. As the spoon gets close to the mouth, the mouth opens and the food goes in - Bingo! Do you really want to have to make those chuffing and zooming noises at every mealtime? Don't you think your child should learn to use a spoon themselves, rather than have an adult do it for them? Once again, this well-intentioned activity is rewarding the behaviour that you don't want: i.e. not eating the food that is there. Don't play that game.

I have also read advice that encourages singing "eating songs" and other such devices to get a child to eat their food. I sympathise with the idea that mealtimes should be happy and positive experiences for all children. But my personal view is that this is for children with real eating problems and disorders. For the rest of us, in my view, singing is not an appropriate activity while trying to eat. It slows everything down and is not conducive to learning to use knives, forks, eating with your mouth closed and so on.

Rule 14: do not "bribe" with puddings or other sweet foods

I cover the nutritional "value" of sweet foods in chapter 6. In summary, consuming sweets, cakes and biscuits – even many of those "children's yoghurts" that are provided by the supermarkets – are simply going to increase the proportion of sugar and fat in your child's diet, without providing much of nutritional value. I don't think that having too many sweet things is good for any child. Equally, I feel that "bribing" a child daily with pudding sets up an uneasy relationship with that type of food. As an adult, it is much easier to avoid less healthy foods if we have not learnt to see them as a reward to ourselves for good behaviour.

The other problem with offering sweet things as reward for eating a main meal is that you are increasing the value of sweets, biscuits, cakes and puddings as a commodity, compared with, say, the peas on the plate waiting to be eaten. You are saying "if you eat the yucky thing, then I will give you the nice thing". But your child and you should want both the peas and the sweet things equally. Ideally, the peas should be the more attractive thing in the long term. The message you need to give to yourself and others is "All the food I give you is tasty and good. Please eat and enjoy it".

You may find that young children will ask for a pudding or other sweet rewards. If they go to a nursery, they are probably being given a pudding with their lunch every day and this may be setting up an expectation that every savoury course is followed by something sweet. I found the most practical thing to do in this situation was to explain why we don't have a pudding after every meal and that chocolates, sweets and deserts are alright to eat sometimes, but not good to have every day. My children understood and were happy with this from a very young age. You are entitled to be in charge and to be the person who knows best. There should be no reason why your child won't accept your judgement on this matter.

In our household, puddings are nowhere near a daily event. We usually have lots of fruit on offer, including tinned varieties which can be brought out as a "pudding" when required. We sometimes buy the sugar-free yoghurts which the children ask for and we make a few fruit-based puddings, such as crumbles. But we hardly ever buy or make things like chocolate puddings, toffee puddings or cakes. Some people have a "treat" jar or tin containing sweets and chocolates to give their children when they have been good or eaten a meal. We don't buy sweets and chocolates. Often a child's party bag will include a bag of chocolate buttons or similar and we keep these for occasional treats. Because the children have not been brought up to eat them, the adults in the house have gradually been "weaned" away from sweet things. So, all round, puddings and sweet things generally are not a big part of our diet.

My personal opinion is that puddings, sweets and chocolates should be limited to only once or twice each week.

Rule 15: eat together whenever you can

Quite a lot of people that I know do not seem to eat meals together more than about once a week. When I went to work in an office it was quite difficult to arrange for us all to eat a meal at the same time in the evenings. What often happened was that the children would get their food as soon as they were brought home from the nursery and then we would eat later. But we always had breakfast together - even if it meant preparing it the night before and getting up a bit earlier. And if one of us was working from home, we would try and eat as a family in the evening. We almost always managed it on a Friday and, at weekends, most meals were together.

Joanna Blythman, in her book "Bad Food Britain", bemoans the fact that so few people eat together and summarises why family meals are a positive thing:

"They strengthen communication between family members and help build relationships on a daily basis: children talk more to parents and this strengthens their linguistic skills, making them more articulate and personable, so giving them an edge in the job market; they learn social skills such as how to share things and listen to other people; they develop good manners. Basic skills, such as learning to use a knife and fork, or holding a simple conversation with an adult, are much less readily acquired by children who eat on their own"[xxiii].

A survey by Cancer Research UK concluded that mealtimes which were regular and at which parents were present were generally healthier. The children ate more fruit and vegetables. The study also emphasised the importance of Mum's and Dad's own consumption habits, as these directly influenced what younger members of the family were eating.

Finally, everyone eating together reduces the burden of work on the person or people who are preparing and cooking food. And going back to the ideas about what babies and toddlers should eat: why shouldn't they eat the same food as you, even if at a slightly different time? If you are having lasagne and salad for dinner, so should your children, once they can chew properly. This is an opportunity for you to reduce the effort required to produce meals and to only cook once for all the people in the house. If the children are eating their tea at 5.30 in the evening, it is still possible for you to eat the same meal at a more civilised time later on.

Rule 16: encourage good table manners

Whatever your personal views on the importance of table manners, there is good reason to establish some basic rules. If your children are sitting with you, you can see what they are eating. If they learn to eat properly and to use a knife and fork they are learning life skills. Staying at the table until everyone is finished is, I feel, part of respecting the person who has cooked the meal.

Some friends of ours never seemed to be able to get their children to sit at the table with the adults when they visited us for meals. Another child I know would refuse to eat what he was given and then, when his mother tried to persuade him, he would simply leave the table. An older child would leave the table without asking and then go to the fridge to help himself to something he fancied.

Leaving the table is the same as a very young child refusing food – it is a form of attention-seeking. My children have done this a few times and I have given them the choice to sit back down or for me to take their plates away. They don't do it any more. If your child does refuse to come back to the table to eat a meal, then you will need to be very firm on the one hand, while ignoring him or her completely on the other hand. Here is what I mean:

Dad: "Joe, please come back and sit down with the rest of us".

Joe: "No".

Dad: "If you come and sit down, you can have your lunch. You cannot have your lunch if you stay over there".

Joe: (no answer).

Dad: "Ok, then".

What Dad must then do is ignore Joe completely. At the end of the meal, if Joe still has not come back to the table, Dad should take his plate away and carry on as usual. By dinner, Joe will almost certainly feel hungry and unlikely to want to spend another mealtime being ignored.

I once came across a child who had developed a habit of rooting in the fridge half-way through a meal. Apart from being quite scandalised that his parents didn't stop him, I couldn't understand why they didn't just move the things he wanted - or stop buying them altogether. No treats or rewards should be given to someone who can't be bothered to wait until everyone else has finished their food. If they have finished a long time before everyone else, then perhaps they need to slow down their eating, anyway.

Here is a list of rules 12 to 16.

12. Make it clear what happens if they eat the food and what happens if they do not – and stick to it
13. Don't make a fuss
14. Do not "bribe" with puddings or other sweet foods
15. Eat together whenever you can
16. Encourage good table manners.

Summary

The most positive start you can give your children as they start learning about food is to give them as much opportunity as possible to try lots and lots of different things to eat.

As you do this, be positive and enthusiastic about food and all the new experiences your child is having. You may need to throw out some of your own assumptions about what babies and toddlers should eat while thinking carefully about how you behave and what you say in relation to food and meals.

You should consistently reward your child for eating and ignore the type of behaviours associated with not eating or being "picky". However, you need to be careful about how you reward your child – you can do this with other things than puddings!

Don't worry if something new is refused. This is normal. But don't be put off by it, either – and do not offer an alternative choice to your child. Keep offering the food and make sure that your child is not substituting meals with snack food.

Be realistic about what your child can eat and, if necessary, start them off with "mini meals". You and your children should always try everything on your plate and then you can always offer more of something that he or she likes as a reward. Make it clear what you expect and what the outcome will be if food is eaten (or not eaten). Ignore the behaviour you do not want and never make a fuss about food being refused.

Don't use sweets and puddings to "bribe" your children, because this sets up an unhelpful psychological relationship with that type of food.

Whenever you can, eat as a family with your children and encourage good table manners.

Having become familiar and applied the rules set out in this chapter you should feel confident that your children are eating a broad range of foods and they are happy with meals and mealtimes. If you feel at any point that some foods are starting to be avoided or meals are becoming stressful then you may have stopped using some of the rules. Remember to be consistent in applying them. You know they work – you just have to make sure you always do and say the same things so that everyone is clear that the food on the plate is there to be eaten.

Summary of the rules for young children and their families

Rule number	The rule
Ground Rules	
1	Get into a routine
2	Give your child as many different things to eat as you can
3	Don't start them off on junk
4	Discard your pre-conceptions and prejudices about what a child should eat
5	Say the right things
6	Reward the behaviour you want and ignore the behaviour you do not want
How to Make Sure They Eat What You Give Them	
7	If food is refused, offer it again at a later time and keep on doing it
8	Never offer an alternative
9	Adapt snack arrangements to maintain an appetite for proper meals
10	Give your child a portion of food that you can reasonably expect them to eat
11	You must always try all the food on your plate
Supporting Strategies	
12	Make it clear what happens if they eat the food *and* what happens if they do not eat the food – and stick to it
13	Ignore the behaviour you do not want – do not make a fuss
14	Do not bribe with puddings or other sweet foods
15	Eat together whenever you can
16	Encourage good table manners

4 WHY ARE OUR CHILDREN GETTING SO PICKY?

Why do so many children seem to control what they eat? I was in the café of the swimming pool recently and overheard the conversation of the family next to us:

Mum: "What would you like to eat? You could have egg and chips, fish fingers and chips or sausage and chips."
Older Boy: "I'd like sausages and chips, please".
Younger Boy: "I want a sandwich".
Mum: "Well I want you to have hot food, because we are not having tea at home".
Younger Boy: "I don't like hot food".
Mum: "Also, you need to choose some vegetables to eat with this. I bet you haven't had any vegetables today?"
Younger Boy: "I want a sandwich. I don't want vegetables".

It went on from there. To me, this seems extraordinary. The children were being offered something which most youngsters would want to eat, yet still this little boy was making a fuss and trying to get something other than his mother had suggested. The whole thing broke down very rapidly into crying and shouting and the poor mum threatening to take them all home. This is not a child making a choice. It is a child manipulating an adult to get their own way, to draw attention to themselves, for whatever reason. In my view, there is no positive "spin" that could be put on what the boy was doing – he was simply attempting to gain control. When I thought about it, I realised that *most* of the children that I know are controlling what they eat and some of them exercise this control *a lot*. If a child is unhappy for a particular reason – for example, if their parents are in the process of a divorce – it is understandable for them to express this in ways which enable them to regain some control of their lives. I think it is up to the parents to try and work out some aspects of their life which they might exert control over without damaging their long-term chances. However, few children who are "difficult" about food appear to have a compelling reason to be like this.

There seem to be lots of children who don't eat fruit. One mother told me that she buys some kind of dried fruit stick in a plastic tube, in order to get her little boy to have some fruit every day.

There are children who have to have the same things for breakfast every day. As an adult, can you imagine being a visitor to someone's house and popping down to the local shops to buy "cornflakes" or "weetabix" for your breakfast because the family didn't have them? Some friends of ours did just that when they found out that the breakfast on offer was fruit and toast. They knew their children wouldn't eat it, so they rushed out for back-up!

I know children who won't eat any green (or any other colour) vegetables, so their parents try and compensate by giving them lots and lots of fruit.

I also know a little boy who basically refuses most food he is offered, because he knows his mother gets upset and angry, or cries.

Again, these are not food choices – these are children who are exerting some kind of control by refusing certain types of food – or all food, if they can get away with substituting meals for snacks. No child will eat everything. No adult will eat everything. I don't really like peanuts in cooking. I will eat them, but I don't really enjoy the taste of them. My sister has always disliked mushrooms and she still avoids them whenever she can. My daughter also dislikes mushrooms, so I never force her to eat more than a spoonful of them. It is pretty normal, then, for an individual to have one or two things that they prefer not to eat. But not fifty things. Not all fruit, or all green things, or anything crunchy. That is nothing to do with food likes or dislikes – it is just a type of behaviour. And I believe that mostly this behaviour is caused by the availability of food in our society and generated by the way in which we, as parents, behave.

But a few – just a few – children, eat most of what they are given. They sit at the table, they use their spoons, knives and forks to the best of their ability and they are happy to try new things with very little fuss or comment. One of my daughter's friends visited on her own, aged four, for the first time. I asked her if she would like to choose what they were having for tea - pasta or jacket potato. What I didn't say was that either of these options would be coming with a mixed lentil and tomato sauce and a side salad. She chose the jacket potato. She didn't make a fuss, or ask what the pudding was, or what was going with the potato. All the children sat properly, ate their food, had some fruit and cake and then went to play in the garden. So why are some children so difficult to please when it comes to food and eating?

Parental perception

With very few exceptions, children will consume the same overall amount of food (calories) every day. However, the time at which they eat and the quantity of food taken in at those times varies enormously[xxiv]. You might have noticed this already. It is perfectly normal for a child to eat lots of food one day and hardly anything the next. You may also have noticed patterns of eating in which your child gobbles up everything in sight for days or weeks on end and then appears to suffer a kind of "slump" in their appetite, reverting to eating less than you were expecting. These variations in eating can lead to some problems of perception about exactly what food your child has taken in.

A friend has always reported to me that her son is a very poor eater and she can barely get food into him. Every mealtime is a struggle, often involving tantrums, kicking and screaming. However, I noticed that although the little boy ate hardly any of what he clearly didn't fancy at mealtimes, he was given many opportunities for snacking. In one instance, having eaten a small bowl of dry cereal for his breakfast, we took him out for the day. He had a banana for his mid-morning snack and then the bread from a sandwich for his lunch – refusing the filling, some salad and a yoghurt. Going back on the train he told my friend he was hungry, upon which she produced two chocolate biscuits from her handbag. Not surprisingly, he ate them!

If you do really feel that your child is not eating enough, then you can check this properly, by keeping a food diary for a few days or a week. Then use the nutritional information in Chapter 6 to assess what is actually being consumed.

I think you will be surprised at exactly how many calories he or she is eating, even though they seem not to want to eat a proper lunch or dinner. You may also be able to assess the quality of the food your child is eating and whether this is a truly balanced diet. You could be preparing very healthy meals, which are regularly being rejected or avoided, in favour of poor-quality (in nutritional terms) snack-time fill-ins.

Parental role models

Are you a "fussy" eater? Are there lots of things you don't like very much? What you eat will affect what your children eat. I suspect you know that already. If you eat healthily, so will the rest of the family - especially if you are the person that is the primary provider of meals in the home.

Someone I know ate main meals consisting of essentially meat, potatoes and onions. No vegetables. No fruit. When the family had children, they all ate together regularly at mealtimes. By the time the boys were six or seven, they had started to copy Dad and it was a real struggle to get them to eat any vegetables at all, despite all the positive efforts of Mum to cook healthy, balanced meals. Fortunately, things have improved and my friend does now eat quite a few vegetables. I have seen him eating peppers, peas and tomatoes, for example. His children eat a fairly balanced range of food, too.

If there are lots of things that you do not like eating, please, *please* start trying them over again. There is research[xxv] that demonstrates that you may have to eat something up to ten times to become accustomed to it and actually enjoy it. But you probably will. And if you choose to eat a wide variety of foods, you are being the best and most positive role model to your children. Research carried out by Cancer Research UK showed that the amount of fruit and vegetables children ate was directly related to what their parents ate[xxvi]. It is really hard to explain why your child should eat his or her lettuce, if you do not have any on your plate.

If you are "picky" about what you eat, I bet there are quite a few things that you haven't eaten since you were a child. The school dinners of the past have much to answer for! The roast beetroot that I eat today bears absolutely no resemblance to the frankly vile vinegar-soaked chunks that I was fed at school, alongside a floppy bit of green lettuce and an under-ripe tomato. I don't think it is even possible to buy food like that any more. And certainly the way we cook things has changed beyond recognition in some cases – think about how cabbage used to be presented. Only the over-70s still cook like that! Go on – try one new thing a week and even if you only enjoy half of those things, you will be helping yourself and your family to a more interesting set of choices for the future.

On the other hand, avoiding all the foods you do not like, combined with foods that your partner won't eat, may leave you with very little to choose from. From now on be positive about trying out new foods or things you don't like.

If you have a poor quality diet, it is best to admit it right now and think carefully about how you need to change your eating habits in order to be the best role model for your children. People who change from eating processed, sugary, salty foods to more fresh food, fruit and vegetables often report that they experience food in a different way. They can taste it more and start to find having a range of flavours and textures interesting. I needn't remind you that a better diet can also mean you lose weight and are generally healthier.

As a parent, I think part of my role is to act as a clear advocate for the right way of eating. One of the most shocking aspects of watching Jamie Oliver's programme about what schoolchildren eat[xxvii], was the attitudes of some of their parents. In particular, I remember the TV chef having debates with individual families about the fact that their child didn't want to eat the new, healthier meals he had devised. Why were these families backing up their children in a situation in which someone was making such an extraordinary effort to improve the quality of what they ate in order to increase overall health? Jamie himself is quite clear about the balance of responsibility:

"At the moment, it all depends on their families. There's no food culture at school. And in lots of families people haven't got time for food and cooking......Whether they're lucky kids with good food at home or not, they should all get decent food at school."

Parental guilt

Society and the way we live our lives has provided us with a whole range of reasons to feel guilty about how our children are brought up. Many of us work full- or part-time and feel that we do not spend enough time with our families. The time that we do spend together is often punctuated by rushed shopping trips, DIY, ironing and housework. We worry about whether our children are learning to walk, talk, count, at the same rate as others. We worry about vaccinations and whether these will harm them. We worry about which school and, then, about whether school is pushing our children too hard. We worry about how much television they watch and the time they spend playing with their computer games. We also worry about what food our children eat.

Compared with many other European countries, people in the United Kingdom have a different relationship with food. We spend far less money on it and less time thinking, preparing, cooking and eating it than the French and Italians, for example. Food is less important to most of us. You may feel guilty about what your toddler is eating and the fact that you cannot get him or her to consume vegetables. But, because of the way our society views meals and eating, it may be that you feel that this is a less important issue than whether your little boy or girl will be able to cope at nursery without you. I believe that this has led to a situation in which parents will "let it go" where the issue of food is concerned. They are too busy, too stressed and feel too guilty about everything. If tackling what their children eat in a positive way means there will be tears and upset, then they are not prepared to go through with that.

If you feel like that – like it is going to be too much to get everyone to eat lots of food – too much of an uphill struggle, then maybe this book is not for you. You have to believe that it would be worth it in the end and changing what they eat now will make the rest of their lives better overall, otherwise there is no point in bothering to apply the rules in the next chapter.

Children in control?

"It's the only thing they have control over". Have you heard that said about why children start to refuse certain foods? The implication is that parents need to be understanding and allow a child this form of expression as part of the development process. Considering how important food is to health and how little insight anyone under the age of about seven will have into this relationship, I am not sure this can be justified. Anyway, are we saying that our children cannot choose what they play with, which DVD they watch, who they become friends with at toddlers club or playgroup? These are all things over which most children have a degree of control and which are not likely to produce any long-term effects on their health. I think that in this instance, as parents, we need to be very clear that we know best. We understand why certain foods are good and why it is of benefit to eat them. We need to be in charge.

I think that all parents worry about whether their child is eating enough and whether what they are eating is the right type of food. But media hype and society's emphasis on being a success at whatever you do, have increased the pressure and the level of anxiety around our children's eating habits. Some mothers and fathers lose confidence and their children pick up on this. The fun starts with a few food items being rejected at mealtimes, and then a few more, until the jam-sandwich scenario can be reached: any food whatsoever that is consumed is a huge relief to the parents, regardless of its nutritional content.

What I want for my children is for them to have choices and a degree of control over what they eat now. But I also need to make sure that the choices they make are from the broadest, widest, healthiest range of food I can possibly get them. I want my children to be able to choose either an apple or a pear and to then find eating that piece of food enjoyable. I don't want to feel at all nervous or anxious about the food my offspring are eating.

Children who manipulate

Children are the best people in the world at getting round their parents, aren't they? In our house, if someone doesn't get their own way with Mum, they will go to Dad and try the same request. This can back-fire - especially if Mum is within earshot! Children who control their food intake to those things they like eating and avoid foods they do not like eating, are often good manipulators. They may be gentle about it -negotiating sweet rewards for good behaviour and thus not feeling hungry when mealtimes come round, so that they can avoid having to eat any nasty vegetables. Or they may be loud and brutish, resorting to crying or floor-kicking tantrums, working themselves up into such a state that they are unable to eat and have to be pacified with a biscuit later on.

There might be a perfectly understandable reason why a parent relinquishes control. A friend had throughout pregnancy suffered very bad morning sickness. She was even admitted to hospital because of her levels of dehydration. When her little boy was born, he didn't put on weight as rapidly as he should have done and his parents were obviously very concerned about this. The problem was soon resolved, however – and her son rapidly caught up with his peers in height and weight. But he never ate breakfast. The morning routine was, get up, try and feed him some breakfast, get ready for walk. By this time, the toddler would be banging on the front door to get out! My friend would put him in the pushchair, walk around town and past the bakery. At which point she would go into the shop and buy her son a sausage roll – which he ate with relish! It never occurred to her to tell the little one that she was going to stop buying him a sausage roll and if he didn't want his breakfast he would have to wait until lunchtime. Her behaviour was driven by her early fears about his weight and the fact he wouldn't eat properly – she was too worried about this to be able to rationalise the fact that she should have re-arranged his routine to ensure he ate breakfast. Maybe if she had started him with a sausage roll first thing she could gradually have moved him on to slightly healthier options, in time.

I think the most effective way in which clever children manage their own consumption habits is when they have the measure of their daily routine and can then pick and choose when and what they eat without too much notice being taken. My little boy developed a rather pronounced milk-drinking habit when he was around a year old. It took me a while to understand that this meant that he often wasn't hungry when the next meal came round. Or that he didn't need to eat the meal in front of him.

Once I had worked out that he was balancing the things he wasn't interested in with milk, I could confidently reduce the amount of milk that he was allowed to drink: when the cup was finished he could have water if he was still thirsty, but no more milk until the end of the meal.

Evolutionary adaptation

Now I have been misleading you a bit, because despite all that I have set out in this chapter, there actually is some evidence that children become more "discerning" about what they eat from about age two onwards. This is thought to be linked to a time when it would be safer and more beneficial to seek out and consume foods which taste sweet or are fatty, because they have more calories and are better for survival. In nature, bitter tastes are often linked to poisons, so it is possible that a child will avoid these as a similar evolutionary tactic[xxviii]. But while the tendency of any child to become fussier as they get older can be understood, it does not follow that this should be allowed to dominate eating habits. One thing that few of us think about is the availability of sweet and fatty foods now – far more than there were when we were all living in caves. What we also know is that children will imitate the eating choices of those people they admire[xxix]. In Mexico, children enjoy the taste of hot food from a very young age. I remember eating curry on toast as a child, because that is what my grandfather had for his tea. My niece, who refused fruit at home, nevertheless copied my own children when she was with them and happily chomped her way through strawberries, raspberries, peaches and any other items on offer.

Again, this supports my view that your role as a positive advocate and eater of lots of different kinds of food is crucially important in determining what your child will choose to eat. If your little boy or girl sees you trying everything, without making any fuss about it, they will be inclined to do the same.

I recently read that as many as one in five children below the age of five years old are what is described as "faddy" about food. For about one third of these children, this behaviour can go on until they are around eight years old[xxx]. But let's face it – much toddler behaviour is "faddy" – it is just part of being that age. And faddiness can be ignored and pretty quickly discouraged by some parents, while others find it much harder to get their children back into "normal" behaviour patterns. What the information about eating problems in children doesn't elucidate is to what extent the so-called "faddy" behaviour is linked to what parents eat, what they say and how they, too behave in relation to food. I know a child who never wants to eat breakfast. His mother, who is a single parent, has resorted in the past to giving him a sausage roll to start his day with. But *she* never has breakfast at home. How can she even start to wonder why this boy is showing solidarity with her by also refusing that meal?

Repeated experience of food increases a child's acceptance of that food[xxxi]. In other words, your influence as a parent will be an important feature of the diet of your children as they grow into adults. Do you remember the story about my daughter and the pasta meal she spat out? I felt had to keep giving it to her because I needed to make sure she would actually grow to like and eat pasta!

Summary

So, are children more "picky" nowadays? I don't think so. There are plenty of grown-ups who are fussy eaters, too. There is more choice for children now. They genuinely don't have to eat their meals because most of them are lucky enough to live in an environment which tends towards over-feeding and this means that they can leave half of what is on their plate and still feel satisfied. They often know that a snack is just a couple of hours away or that they will be given a "treat" such as cake or biscuits at the end of every meal. They can hang out for that, if they want.

I think that some parents feel such pressure to feed their children that they have lost the confidence to apply some common sense. They find it impossible to say "no" to what their child asks for - even when that same child has refused the food in front of them. And the whole debate about nutrition can blind us to the simple fact that when someone is hungry, they will eat. It is only when an individual is not hungry that picking and choosing becomes an option.

The main things that influence whether a child will choose to eat a certain food are the actions and behaviour of their parents and other important carers. It goes without saying that if you feed your children a limited, bland range of relatively unhealthy foods, then that is the type of food they will want to eat as they grow up. If you make sure you provide a good range of food, that you eat the same food and you are clearly positive about eating a fresh, balanced diet, then the younger members of the family will be inclined to eat in the same way.

5 PRACTICAL ADVICE FOR THE OLDER CHILD

This chapter is for parents of children from about the age of four who may be just about to start school or already at school, right up to early teenage years. Basically, if your child is capable of negotiating with you, the rules that you should apply are in this section of the book. However, you should see this as a supplement to chapter 3. Almost all of the rules that work with younger children will also work with older children and the main principles about you as food advocate, key role model and provider of healthy options apply to all ages of children. If you have turned straight to this section, you will find it helpful to go back and read chapters 3 and 4 and then come back to this point.

Whenever I visit teashops, cafes and lunchtime restaurants, I am amazed at what children eat – and what their parents let them eat. But I am also amazed at how unhappy everyone seems to be as they sit round their plates of chips, burgers, beans and sodas. Surely, if we took a more – say – Italian or French attitude to our food, everyone would be sitting there (for some time) discussing the food and actually enjoying it!

I have heard parents saying things like "Adam is so difficult with food. He won't eat any vegetables at all. But it's too late to do anything about it now." From my own experience, I know that this is not true. I have watched how other children have improved in what they eat as they get older and have had close and regular contact with a child in my own home, who was a very picky eater. From the age of about five, he ate hardly any vegetables and certainly no foods that he had not tried before in his own home. But, over time, this little boy has learned that what he is given to eat is to be eaten. He still doesn't always eat what is on his plate, but he is many times better than he used to be. He will always try foods properly and understands that he cannot "get away" with leaving piles on his plate, or under his fork. And he knows that it is down to him whether he gets second portions of what he likes or maybe a pudding.

The other source from which you can see that people have changed what appear to be entrenched attitudes, lifestyles and eating habits, including those of their children, is television shows. While they rely largely on a shock element to provoke some action in the people involved and gloss over much of the hard work and – I assume – arguments about what the family will eat, the participants themselves are able to explain how they have managed to change in order to assure themselves a much better long-term standard of health and life.

Never Too Late

It is never too late to ensure a child chooses, eats and enjoys good food. This chapter is for those of you who have older children who may have become difficult to please, or who refuse more foods than they decide to eat. If mealtimes and eating out are stressful, now is the time to change things. And don't worry – you have a lot more influence and control than you may think. It is certainly not too late to tackle what the people in your family eat – no matter how old your children are.

If you are reading this book and your children are already past the age of about five or six, I believe you may be facing a challenge of changing some fairly entrenched family-wide behaviour. This might include a range of issues, including fussiness, food refusal and an unwillingness to eat anything unfamiliar and/or healthy. If this is the case, for you to simply start applying the rules I set out in this book is likely to meet with some resistance. I recommend that once you have decided your action plan for tackling the range of issues you face, you sit everyone down and tell them in advance exactly what you intend to do. Remember, you will be consistent and firm and each member of the family needs to understand how their own behaviour will have to change in order to conform to the new rules of the household. Alongside rule number 17 I give an example of how to get everyone "signed up" to a particular course of action. Don't worry if, to start with, no-one wants to go along with you or change their behaviour – you will still be able to apply your principles.

Ground Rules - Revision

Here are some examples of the way in which the rules I have already set out can be adapted for slightly older children. The numbers are the same as in chapter 3, so that you can reference back to the relevant rules in the earlier sections of the book.

<u>Rule 5: say the right things</u>

Remember to use the right language when talking about food. "That looks good" is better than "what is that?", for example. Being positive about food will also help you to feel positive when you try new things. This is much more important than many of us realise. Think about how you encourage your children to think optimistically about things that are coming up – how they will do in their tests, what fun Sports Day will be, how nice it will be to visit Granny at the weekend. The way you think about something in advance affects how you then experience that thing when it happens. Remember, also, to say to yourself, "I enjoy trying new foods and usually like them".

Rule 6: reward the behaviour you want and ignore the behaviour you do not want

Be pleased and happy when food is eaten, but if it is not, don't have a tantrum, don't cry, don't let them know you care that they have left what is on their plate. Move on to the next thing.

Rule 7: if food is refused, offer it again at a later time and keep on doing it

My father was an advocate of the "give it back to them for their next meal" approach to food refusal. Which once resulted in my then three-year-old sister being given the same plate of cold broad beans three times in a row. She still doesn't like broad beans very much, and who could blame her? I don't think this is an effective way to engender a positive view of mealtimes. Still, the principle is that you may need to try a particular food more than once – indeed, up to ten times – before you come to accept and like it. So even if your child is adamant that they do not like, say, pears, please don't throw all the pears in the bin! Continue to give them pears as and when you feel like it and make sure they keep trying a small piece. In time, they will almost certainly come to like them.

My husband didn't like green cabbage, celeriac, sweetcorn, aubergine, chick peas, lentil dhal, raw tomatoes and many other things that he now happily eats and actually enjoys. What he likes about the meals we eat is the variety and lack of repetition. If you keep on working at the range of what your family eats, you should find you are never bored by the meals that you share.

Rule 8: never offer an alternative.

Rule number eight may be harder with an older child. It says that if your child won't eat what they are given, then you just take the food away and that is the end of the mealtime. Let's face it, a baby or toddler may cry when you take the plate away, but within minutes they will have forgotten the incident and be happily playing with teddy. Children from the age of about four rapidly develop that talent euphemistically known as "pester power". They know that you have put eight of their favourite chocolate biscuits in the cupboard. Or that there are some oven chips in the freezer. They will helpfully suggest one of these options in preference to what is on their plate! By all means, agree that one of these "treat" items could be provided after the meal or as part of the next one. But make it clear that they will first have to eat everything that is in front of them right now.

If you remember the section about how a child learns, being consistent and always keeping to the no alternative rule means that you never fall into the trap of rewarding your child for pestering you, whining, sulking or whatever other tactic they may employ to try and get their own way.

Rule 10: give your child a portion of food that you can reasonably expect them to eat

The principle behind this rule is that you want to be able to reward your child for eating all of what is on their plate. Therefore, whether your child is five or thirteen, you can achieve this by starting off with really small "mini meals" as described in chapter 3. Using these to gradually increase the range of food that is eaten is a good strategy to ensure more things are consumed and enjoyed as time goes on. You may find that your child moans at you for not giving him or her enough of their favourite foods, but please do use this tactic if you need to. You give a small meal and when it is completely finished, your child can have more of whatever they like.

Rule 11: you must always try all the food on your plate

Remember, you only need to eat a teaspoonful of any particular food for you to have properly experienced its taste, texture and other features. For an older child, this rule fits well with the "mini meal" approach because you are simply emphasising that the amount that has to be eaten is really very small. There is no pressure to eat it, but there shouldn't be anything else on offer if your child refuses to comply.

Rule 12: make it clear what happens if they eat the food *and* what happens if they do not eat the food – and stick to it

Be courageous! Tell your child what reward (if any) they will receive if they eat their meal. Tell them that if they do not eat it, there will be nothing else to eat until tea-time / the morning. Be clear, then act. Do not give in. Do not promise an alternative. Do not react to tears, tantrums or other behaviour which is designed to make you feel bad. Keep it in proportion: did you ask them to eat an entire plateful of cabbage? – No. Did you tell them you were going to give them the meal again at tea-time? – No. Probably, all you asked them to do was to eat one mouthful of vegetables. There is no good reason for your child to have refused to do this or to do now whatever they are doing. Walk away, if you can, and think about something else until it is time for the next meal.

Rule 13: ignore the behaviour you do not want – do not make a fuss

See the previous rule. You are not the cause of any bad behaviour. You are not the reason your child is refusing to eat their meal. From the age of three or four onwards, you can be certain that children are able to choose whether to eat what they are given or not. If they decide not to eat something, that is up to them. You should already have made it clear that there is nothing else to eat until the next meal. You do not need to react if, after a reasonable amount of discussion and explaining what you would like, they still refuse to eat what is on their plates. Just take it away and go and do something else.

How did we get here?

Here is another story. I was collecting my daughter from the nursery one day, when I overheard a conversation between one of the members of staff and a parent. It went like this:

Carer: "He didn't eat any of his main course at lunch today".
Mum: "What was it?"
Carer: (checks clipboard) "Um, tuna pasta bake with carrots and sweetcorn".
Mum: "But you had fish pie yesterday".
Carer: (Flips pages over and checks again) "Er, yes".
Mum: "He doesn't like fish".

Oh dear. He doesn't like fish. So, he doesn't like tuna sandwiches, fish fingers, fish pie (obviously), baked salmon, kippers, fish cakes, prawn salad? This child has decided, at the age of two, that he dislikes all fish.

Then I thought to myself "no – that's not it......it's his parents". Either *they* don't like fish, or they have responded to his eating habits in such a way that they have set up a pattern whereby he refuses to eat fish. When he has pulled a face at something they have not offered it to him again. When he has left all of a fish finger, they have crossed it off the list of foods to try him with. He has pushed a tuna sandwich off his plate, but they have given him his yoghurt anyway because they thought he was still hungry. These responses, or a combination of these and some other behaviours, have resulted in a child of two who won't eat fish pie for lunch.

However good your parenting skills are and however happy you are with other aspects of family life, somehow a situation has been reached in which your child or children are controlling the food that you prepare and cook for them. This may mean that you are cooking more than one meal during the evening. You could be cooking for everyone separately. You may be feeding the children the sort of food that you, personally, wouldn't dream of eating: fish fingers, cheap sausages, frozen, packaged pizzas and gelatinous, additive-laden pots of sweet puddings.

Why are you doing this? Is it because you can't be bothered, or feel you do not have the time, to cook a family meal? Or is it because everyone argues about what you try and feed them, when you do give them all the same thing?

I have a friend with a little boy who doesn't like vegetables. She works almost full-time and well over the part-time hours she is contracted to work by her employer. She often feels guilty about the fact that her son is at the nursery all day almost every day. When he refuses his tea or part of his tea, she still gives him his yoghurt. He gets upset if she doesn't and she finds it too hard to deal with how this makes her feel.

Lots of children and teenagers use food as a means of manipulating and controlling their parents. They understand that this is a potential weak point. Parents feel guilty about being at work or otherwise too busy for their children. They are anxious to ensure that their children eat the right foods and avoid less healthy things. They worry about whether young children are eating enough. For various reasons, many of us find the processes of eating, preparing and cooking food stressful. We react emotionally to the whole subject and therefore it is no wonder that perfectly sensible people find it difficult to behave in a way that sets clear boundaries and rules and leads to everyone eating the same things, at the same time. And eating it all up.

Back to Proper Meals

Rule 17: one meal, one mealtime

What many families appear to do is to try and have an inexhaustible supply of every kind of food that their child eats. They let the children decide what they want for their breakfast, lunch and tea. They have five different kinds of cereal; three versions of the oven chip; four flavours of fruit squash and no room in their freezers for any vegetables apart from the ubiquitous pea!

They also cook or prepare more than one type of food for every mealtime. Maybe shepherd's pie with vegetables for Mum and Dad, but with chips for someone else, because they don't like the carrots and someone else just has beans on toast.

If this, or a version of it, is happening in your house, you need to take a stand. You need to make sure that it is you, the parents, who are in charge of what everyone eats and when. You should not have to prepare two, three or four different meals to accommodate the various tastes and preferences of the people who live with you.

Furthermore, the people – adults and children - in your house should respect both food itself and the processes related to producing food on their plates. There seems to be a belief among many people that food and eating are almost non-essential parts of our lives. Whereas I believe that they are vitally important. Meals should be healthy and nourishing. They should be enjoyed. This enjoyment should be shared and both children and adults need to participate fully at mealtimes by being there and by sharing family conversation.

I may be rather old-fashioned, but I also feel there is too little respect paid to the people or person in the house who takes charge of buying and cooking food. For many of us, food preparation involves opening a packet of food to be microwaved or popped in the oven, maybe alongside a bag of salad or some frozen vegetables. But even this level of effort is barely acknowledged by our offspring. If your children think that a meal takes five minutes to make, then how much of a shock are they going to get as adults when they have to think about cooking food for their own families? When you spend two hours preparing the Sunday lunch, does anyone else get involved? Or do they make themselves scarce, in case they have to help? When was the last time someone said "thank you" to you for a meal that you cooked?

From now on the food that you cook should be what everyone eats. No more discussion of what everyone wants for the meal – you decide. No more putting the plate on the table and then seeking out other types of food and morsels in the fridge because what you have offered is refused. No more tantrums because the dinosaur shapes weren't in stock in the supermarket and you had to get alphabet ones instead. Take control.

What this rule means is that there will be a single mealtime, which everyone should participate in. Food will not be served at any other time. The food that is on offer is all that there is to eat.

Now you are asking "How do I make this happen?". For children from the age of about four or five, you need to start with an appeal to their better natures and their loyalty to you. Organise a family meeting around the kitchen table and tell everyone what the issue is: perhaps lots of time spent on cooking various types of food, maybe not enough healthy food being eaten, extra work, anxiety and stress for the people making meals, the need to realise that there is someone who is doing all this work and that it is not being appreciated etc. Your issue may just be that your two children won't eat vegetables. Tell them you have decided that these problems can be addressed in part by individual members of the family accepting that all of you should eat the same food. This is not going to be negotiable at this point, but anyone can contribute ideas for healthy meals that they think everyone will enjoy eating.

Make it clear when this new regime will start. It might also be worth drawing up a list of the rules which you will be applying – i.e. one meal choice only, no alternatives, nothing else if a main course is not eaten and trying everything on the plate. Then agree how you will reward your children for their cooperation. For example, by spending some time doing something as a family that they enjoy, such as going to the park, the cinema, swimming or bowling.

Refer to the agreement when things get tough, but do not give in. Remember that you have the right to time for yourself and to a minimal amount of stress. Short-term, there may be tears, tantrums and grief. Remind yourself that things will get better and that when they are you will never have to go back to the bad old days of multiple meals, poor quality food and stressful mealtimes.

Remember, also, rule number 8, which say that you should **never offer an alternative**. As soon as alternatives are offered, you have broken the "not negotiable" rule. If one of the children is refusing to eat their cabbage, for instance, you cannot suggest that they try a bit of cauliflower, instead. You need to be clear, refer to your agreement and ask them to please try the cabbage. If they do not want it, once they have tried it, that is fine, but there isn't anything else available for them to eat.

Rule 18: avoid the pitfall of grazing

When we went to visit my mother-in-law once, my niece and nephew were there too. All of the children are about the same age and they were quite a handful together in one house. After a couple of days I noticed something. They were all doing what I call "grazing". Whenever they wanted some attention, or were a bit bored, they would cluster round their Granny, saying they were hungry. She would find them a snack - maybe some raisins or a breadstick. Perfectly healthy things for them to eat. But they kept on going back and saying they were hungry, so that the day became one long, drawn-out eating session. At lunch and tea time they just picked at what was on their plates and left most of it. We had to ask my mother-in-law not to give the children anything except at mealtimes.

Many parents seem to carry a constant supply of snacks with them. An ammunition store of food options for those times when their offspring are so hungry they cannot go on. Naturally enough, if a child has not eaten much or any of its lunch, he or she is likely to be hungry half-way through the afternoon. But haven't you already explained the situation to them? You told them that if they decided not to eat what was on their plate that there would be nothing else until tea-time. You cannot provide a let-out clause of a banana at 3pm, because you will not be being consistent. The more firmly you adhere to your own rules, the faster your children will understand that mealtimes are for eating. Rationally, however upset your child appears to be, he or she is not going to faint from hunger before tea arrives. However tough this appears to be, remember that you earlier made them a perfectly good meal, which they chose not to eat. If you give them a snack now, they might choose not to eat the next meal you produce and so on. Of course, if everyone has eaten their lunch and you are in the park on a sunny day, there is no reason at all why you can't each enjoy an ice cream.

If you are going to stick with the "one meal, one mealtime" rule, you will also need to be aware of the other ways that children can get round this. They will certainly try. I have already mentioned snacks and how these can be subtly substituted for full meals by discerning youngsters. Teenagers, who often have some financial resources and therefore more control over snack food options can be much harder to manage. You could suggest that you suspend money for snacks, in favour of them taking something from the fruit bowl and fridge in the mornings. Fortunately, schools are becoming a great ally in the healthy eating battle. Because they no longer sell sweets and chocolates on site and they request parents not to let their children bring such foods to school, the opportunity for them to eat junk is much less.

Rule 19: chuck out the junk

For older children at home, if you have already started along the path of bags of crisps, biscuits and those stretchy "cheese" things that some children seem to so enjoy, now would be a good time to revert back to a big bowl of fruit, plain oat biscuits and a pot of humous or yoghurt dip. Before you remove all of your family's favourite snack foods, here are some words of advice.

If you have your own snack food weaknesses, you should either kick the habit at the same time or at least carry out your indulgence at times when no-one else can see you – such as when the children are in bed. It will not be easy to maintain your position or your principles if your offspring catch you munching a bag of crisps half-way through the afternoon.

We have some good friends with two children. The parents are quite concerned about what the boys eat, but feel it is too late to do anything about it. We have never eaten a home-cooked meal at their house. They always get a take-away – even for a midday meal it will be pizza, accompanied by onion rings, battered and deep-fried cheese and never any salad. Pudding is invariably cake or chocolate. While they are clearly aware of what the family diet should be, they appear to like and enjoy the food they buy and seem to have no will to make any real change.

When you are grasping the nettle and eliminating junk food habits from your household, you should tell everyone beforehand what you are doing and why. Whatever you do, don't agree to negotiate for any extra special treats to be kept "on the menu" (or in the kitchen cupboard). Absolutely do not promise the favourite snack foods themselves as a reward for going a whole week without them – or you will never break the junk food cycle. The best thing you can do for the health of yourself (if you are a junk-food consumer) and your family is not to hide the food – just throw it away. And when it is all disposed of, don't buy any more.

Finally, try and get everyone involved in coming up with some healthy alternatives, such as the ones I have mentioned above. Older children may well have been introduced to various ideas at school or at other people's houses, so ask them for their contributions.

Rule 20: increase the range of food that you eat

I have a friend who doesn't eat curry. That's ok – she can have a pizza. She doesn't like rice, or tomatoes, or sweetcorn. She won't eat most types of fish. She wouldn't eat a piece of home-made lemon meringue pie if you gave it to her. Quite frankly, I can't be bothered to remember the things she doesn't eat, so I don't invite her round at mealtimes. I am happy to go to any restaurant she chooses, of course. She usually chooses pizza places.

Do you feel that every mealtime is constrained by a huge list of things that the children won't eat? Does your little boy or girl absolutely refuse to eat anything green, or red, or "mushy", or crunchy? Is every mealtime a nightmare, with noise, tears or tantrums? Or do you feel that you are just giving the children the same things over and over again, because it is easier to do this than to try and get them to eat things they don't like?

Has your child come home from school complaining that there was nothing for them to eat at lunchtime (even though there are three choices every mealtime). Or have you already started to send them with a packed lunch after they pestered you for weeks about it?

In this section I want to explain the steps to getting your child or children to gradually extend and increase the range of food that he or she eats. This will result in more freedom for you in the food that you can offer them – which means less time worrying about whether you can get to the supermarket to buy the only brand of fish cakes that they will all eat. You will be able to make sure they eat more healthy food. And you can send them to school knowing that they *will* eat something for lunch and it may even include some vegetables. Few of us really know what our children eat for school lunch, but we want to have some faith that they will choose something like what they would eat at home. It follows that if you know they have a reasonable range of foods that they will eat at home, you can be fairly confident that they will probably eat similar types of food at school.

The first step for tackling this issue is a discussion with your child or children about food. If they are at school, they may have already been talking about food and healthy eating. They could have been involved in a project about agriculture and what happens to the things that are grown. Anyway, from a young age, children are given quite clear messages about what is healthy to eat and what is not. There are even television programmes which encourage very young children to cook and which also talk about healthy food choices. What you may find, if you open this conversation, is that your children know as much or more about healthy eating as you do!

Recently, my children have started telling our friends and other family members if they are eating unhealthy food. I was in a café a while ago and my daughter told the lady next to us that giving her child a hot chocolate and a muffin was not very healthy! Needless to say, we left quite quickly after that.

Get your children to explain what a healthy diet is, or talk it through with them. Then ask them what the consequences of an unhealthy diet are: being overweight and possibly unhappy as a result, not having good teeth, not being able to go to the toilet (children are bizarrely concerned about this) and not being very well when you are a grown-up, among other things. Ask your child about what they eat every day. It may help to keep a food diary for a few days, because you can count how many portions of various types of food they have eaten. Is it healthy? Why is/isn't this meal healthy? Why didn't they choose the healthy option at school? Your aim in having this conversation is to make it clear to your son or daughter that deciding that lots of foods are not nice to eat makes it much, much harder to be healthy. And they already know why that is not a good thing.

Then explain what action you are going to take to help your child eat more healthy foods. Tell him or her that you are going to start all over again with lots of foods and try them out together. I bet you can hear the moans and complaints already! The rules will be that everyone eats the same things and everyone tries everything. You will all be learning about how things taste at the same time.

Then you need to put this into practice, by re-introducing those foods that have been removed from the family menu. Ignore your current knowledge about what your children like or do not like and simply present them with normal meals, with appropriate accompaniments. Just because one person doesn't like tomatoes doesn't mean they will be excluded from meals in future. Use tactics such as mini meals to make sure that all foods are tried again, even if they are things that individuals do not enjoy. Make sure you say the right things (rule number 4), think positively and ignore bad behaviour.

Don't be put off by the "I don't like that" tactic. Both of my children have tried this. I call it pre-emptive sabotage: they start off by making you believe they won't like it or won't eat it and you are immediately on the defensive, worrying about the scene that might be about to happen. Just ignore this and tell them that they still have to try it – because they haven't had it cooked this way before, or because you have made it specially for everyone to try together – any reason will do, but they have to eat some. Assume that, despite what they say, they have never actually eaten this food and ask them to go ahead.

If you want to work in a reward element as you try new things, you could draw up a family list of all the foods to be "tackled" and tick them off as you go along, allowing a treat for every five ticks.

My husband, as you know, has gradually increased the range and variety of all sorts of foods that he would never previously have looked at, let alone eaten. He has persevered with many tastes and textures that he really didn't enjoy, because he wanted to be able to eat well and healthily. He also wanted to be a good role model to the children. He admits that he does not feel that the way he was "allowed" to avoid many foods as a child was a good thing at all. I respect him hugely for the efforts he has made to broaden his diet and I believe that your family – and especially your children – will likewise respect and agree with your decision to get everyone to eat more foods.

In order to get back to proper meals, start with the rules in this section:
1. One meal, one mealtime.
2. Avoid the pitfall of grazing.
3. Chuck out the junk.
4. Increase the range of food that you eat.

Managing Avoidance

<u>Rule 21: limit meals to a reasonable length of time</u>

Protracted meals can be pretty trying. Don't get me wrong - a long lunch or dinner around the table with family and friends is one of my favourite social events. But I have a boredom threshold of about twenty minutes when sitting at the table with a child who has been picking away at a main course for ages. While this is going on, the rest of us have sat and watched, encouraged and threatened the little one to please finish their food. I think that this is a form of food refusal. In these circumstances, my view is that the food is surplus to requirements and the best approach is to wrap up the meal in whichever way seems appropriate. Here is an example:

Mum: "Josh, are you going to eat that food?"
Josh: (no answer).
Mum: "You know I said that you could have a yoghurt? Well you can, if you eat that up now. But you need to be quick, please."
Josh: "Ok."
(After three minutes)
Mum: "You haven't eaten a single mouthful since I last spoke to you. Are you going to eat it?"
Josh: "I *am*. Leave me alone!"
Mum: "Well, ok, you have four minutes. I am going to put the timer on and if you have finished by the time it buzzes, you can get a yoghurt out. But if you haven't then that is the end of dinner."
Josh: (still poking food around on plate) "Arh, Mum!"
Mum: (ignores him) "Ok, four minutes on the buzzer...."
(After four minutes)

Mum: "Josh, I am taking this away now, because I need to get on with things. Please will you go and get your school bag so I can put your drink and snack in for tomorrow."

The problem is, of course, that you really want your child to eat the food, so you need to give them enough opportunity to do this. And some children are just slower at eating. My little boy can string out a piece of toast for twenty minutes, so imagine how long lunch can take. Remind yourself that taking significantly longer than everyone else is really just another form of food refusal. And remember rule number twelve, which is to make it clear what happens if they eat the food *and* what happens if they do not eat the food – and stick to it. So you are simply changing the condition to one which is "please will you eat the food in the time I have asked you to." As long as they have tried everything that is on the plate, it does not matter if they don't finish it all. If they are hungry later, they will eat more at their next meal. So the steps you must take are to decide how long it is reasonable for a meal to take and then remove the plate when that time is up. As a guide, I suggest that a reasonable time is no more than twenty-five minutes for any course or no longer than fifteen minutes after everyone else has finished the food on their plate.

One other way to make sure that meals are eaten within a reasonable timeframe is to use the mini meal approach. Once the small portion has been eaten, you can decide how much more to give your child and whether this is purely a case of him or her just not being hungry at this particular mealtime.

Rule 22: organise meals to ensure that the rejected foods are eaten

Well, here I am at the dinner table and once again my son has eaten all of his pizza and left the salad on the side of his plate. I have told him there is nothing else to eat and he is completely unconcerned because, a) he had a banana and a fairy cake (big mistake) when he got home from school and he isn't that hungry and, b) he is not very interested in the healthy yoghurt that I have offered him for after the main course. This is all part of a trend in which he willingly munches all sorts of things but somehow always manages to avoid the green salads and vegetables that I encourage everyone to eat.

In France it is fairly common to eat salad as a course before anything else, often followed by vegetables and then finally a meat course. It is also standard to eat it all with lots of white bread, but I will gloss that fact over for the purposes of the point I am about to make! It is that you can re-organise mealtimes to make sure that the important things like salads are actually being eaten. It may feel a little strange to have a small plate of peas and beans in front of you while your lamb chops are still grilling, but if you are really having problems getting everyone to try beans, then do it.

You might need to combine this approach with rule 8 – no alternatives, rule 10 – a portion that you can expect them to eat (including, if necessary, going back to "mini meal" –sized portions) and rule 11 – always trying what is on your plate. Basically, you should be giving the message that this is an important part of the meal you have cooked. It is here to be eaten. Once you have eaten it, we will move on to the next course. If you do not eat it, your meal is over.

As I suggest above, you don't need to make a big deal of this. You may decide to start with really small portions of your new vegetable/salad course. But the key thing is to be very firm that it needs to be eaten if the remainder of the meal is to be made available. I used this approach very effectively with a little girl who would eat no salad or fruit and after three meals she "got it" and started to eat the tiny portions of these which I was offering her. One day we had peas and beans, followed by fish cakes; the next day was salad and then pizza and another day we had sweetcorn as a starter before the main course.

One huge benefit of eating this way, which probably contributes to the legendary health of the Mediterranean way of life – is that it is really easy to make sure that my children are eating enough vegetables and salads, especially during the week when it can be hard to know how many of their five-a-day they have consumed while at school. There is nothing written down that says how you need to order a meal. My children think it is normal to have fruit or salad at the beginning of a meal. Be confident and remain in charge: if you decide that a tin of sweetcorn is first on today's menu, who is going to argue with that?

Rule 23: exclude disruptive influences

If not before, certainly when your offspring start school they will want their friends to come home with them. And this, of course, means that you will end up feeding children other than your own. Like most parents, I "play safe" when I am expecting young visitors and offer something like pizza, spaghetti bolognaise or a jacket potato. Even with these relatively unchallenging food options, some children that have been to visit have refused what is on their plate, leaving me with a bit of a dilemma: should I treat these children as if they were my own and not offer them anything else, or should I provide them with something which they will eat, regardless of my principles and any future arguments that might arise with my children?

Here is what I have done when a visiting child has refused food: First, I have told them that in our house we always try what we have on our plates. This is if the children have not beaten me to it – like all youngsters they are not slow to point out when someone is not conforming to their idea of how things should happen! If the child then eats some of what they have, they can have something else. If they do not eat any of the food, I then offer them a) a piece of fruit and/or b) a piece of bread and butter. And then I explain what I have done when their parents arrive to pick them up. Most mums and dads are absolutely fine with this approach and often rather embarrassed that food has been a problem during the visit. I have not yet had any parent berate me for sending their child home hungry and I have not noticed future invitations to tea being refused. However, I have to confess to having worked hard to dissuade my own children from re-inviting "problem eaters" to our house!

It is not my responsibility to ensure that the children of the local community all eat as broad a range of healthy food as my own do. But I do see it as part of my role to avoid bringing into our home people who will disrupt family mealtimes, which are generally a harmonious and happy affair! I want to protect our approach to eating and food and will take steps to do this as necessary.

The other side of the peer pressure coin can, of course, be a lever to get your child to eat better. I am sure you will have noticed that irritating habit of otherwise "picky" children who eat everything on their plate when they visit their best friend's house. It can be hard for a six-year-old to retreat from the unavoidable truth that at Alice's house yesterday she ate a pear, even though she says she doesn't like them. I think it is perfectly acceptable to remind your children if they have eaten foods elsewhere that they are refusing to consume at home.

When I was a child I aspired to those icing-covered, square "french fancy" cakes and "toast toppers", because that is what my best friend had for her tea. All I can conclude is that my parents didn't encourage this relationship, because I now wouldn't know where to find a toast topper in the supermarket, let alone how to cook it.

Finally, you may need to be aware that "disruptive" influences can take many guises. A friend told me that she had adopted some of my ideas with her little boy and was finding that his eating habits had improved. One day, however, after having told him that he couldn't have anything else when he refused to eat his tea, she discovered her husband feeding her son a "jaffa cake!"

Rule 24: manage shock tactics as food refusal

Very young children can become adept at manipulating their parents with tears and tantrums. Older children have a different armoury of tools at their disposal. Being aware of some of these will help you to anticipate them and manage them if they arise.

To my dismay, both of my children went through a short phase of spitting out their food. What they do is either to drop it out of their mouth onto their plate, or to audibly say "pah!" and spit it with some force. Spitting is disgusting. Unless food is "off" or contains a foreign object (such as a hair or fishbone) there is no excuse for it. As soon as they spit, tell them how you feel about the behaviour and ask them to eat another mouthful of the food. They don't have to eat all of the portion you have given them, but they must chew and swallow at least a teaspoonful.

There are two reasons for making them do this. First, they might be trying to avoid the food and this is not acceptable – they should know that they always have to try something, which means chewing and swallowing it. Second, this may be a reaction to a particular aspect of the food – such as a slimy or chewy texture or a bitter taste. If you accept this and allow them not to eat the thing they do not like, then you are establishing an opt-out for things that are similarly slimy, chewy or bitter. So, if your child spits out aubergine, because it is slimy, he might then spit out mango, which feels the same in his mouth.

The second of the above reasons for being very firm about this behaviour leads to one other point, which is not to discuss at any length the reason why your child spat out their food. You don't want to start a negotiation about whether or not the food is "horrid", "nasty" or whatever other adjective he or she can come up with. I doubt if you have gone out of your way to produce a meal that is in any way horrid or nasty, so that is not a conversation you need to have, is it?

If a young child refuses to try a further mouthful, or if the spitting happens again, then you may have no choice except to terminate the meal immediately. This is not a punishment. But you cannot accept this type of behaviour. Don't make a fuss. Explain that if they do not try the food you will have to take the rest of the meal away, but if they do try it, there will be more of what they like or a piece of fruit/a sticker/some television and see if that works. Finally, if that, too has failed just take the plate away.

You will have to try this food again within a few days. You may feel it is worth telling your son or daughter that this will happen, so that they know you have not allowed them to "get away" with spitting. They need to understand that they will not be able to avoid it and it would be better if they tried it, got used to it and could eat it like everyone else.

When offering the same food again, you will be the best judge of how to handle the situation. However, I think it is perfectly reasonable for you to offer a small treat for carrying out your request to try the food again – maybe that you will spend some time doing something with your daughter or son later on. Your aim is to achieve compliance and harmony, not a full-blown battle within the family and you certainly don't want anything to escalate so that it does become a problem.

If an older child – from about the age of seven or eight upwards – starts to spit food out, you may need to think about what this behaviour means. Food aversions, which are covered briefly on the next page, usually arise before this age. Therefore spitting is almost certainly something that your child has decided to do. It is a behaviour that they have judged will shock you. They think that it will make sure that you do not give them that food to eat – now or in the future. It is the equivalent of simply deciding to refuse that particular food.

Set out a mini meal which is one teaspoon of all of its components. This might be a teaspoon of mashed potato, a teaspoon of chicken, a teaspoon of carrots and a teaspoon of the thing your child is refusing to eat/spitting out – perhaps courgette. The size of the meal is in proportion to the issue. All your child needs to do is to eat the mini meal and then he or she can have as much as she likes of the remainder of the meal. Even if this is all mashed potato and chicken and not a single mouthful more of carrots and courgettes. All that matters is that your child has tried and eaten one mouthful of the previously rejected food. This should be a "win-win" situation: if your child eats the mouthful of the food that they allegedly do not like, then you are happy and they will get to eat a full meal and not be hungry. They might choose not to eat the mini meal, however. In this case, they will have made the choice to be hungry and to remain so until the next main meal of the day. I have used this approach on older children and they soon get bored of being hungry and/or of being offered the mini meal version of every course. They rapidly move to eating the tiny portion quickly, at which point you can increase the portion sizes of everything, including the food they say they do not like. Even the most stubborn child will get the message about food refusal within a month.

I have also seen children "gagging" on food. To me, this is the same as spitting, although it is much more exploitative and manipulative of the poor parents who have to watch such behaviour. If your child starts to do this, ask yourself: "Is this a normal response to food, or are they doing it simply as a way of refusing the food and to discourage me from trying to offer it again?" If you let your child avoid a food completely because he or she is apparently about to vomit, what are you rewarding him or her for doing? How long will it be before the tactic is brought into play again? How long before you are back to square one, with only eight meal options available for the whole family to happily eat together? Once again, try to put this into perspective. What harm can he or she come to if you insist that he/she chews and swallows a single mouthful of cabbage? All members of the family need to understand that just because a food is refused once does not mean it will never re-appear on the table. Tackle gagging incidents in the same way you would handle spitting (see above).

You may wish to suggest that the best policy will be for your child to eat it now because in the long term this will help them to enjoy as many types of food as possible.

However old they are children do not like to be ignored. I have a child who has visited my house regularly since he was about four. From about the age of six he started refusing to eat a variety of foods – mostly unfamiliar things. I told him that he would only be getting small portions of food and then he could have what he wanted. For a while that worked, but then he started gagging on things he really didn't want to eat. We decided to completely ignore this behaviour: we were positive and enthusiastic if the food was eaten – even if it had been accompanied by noises and faces - but if it was not, we said nothing and simply cleared the plate away. This may seem harsh – even cruel – but because I was consistent and the message was always unequivocal, there was no argument to be had. Within a few visits the behaviour had stopped because it received no positive reinforcement.

Food phobias are not common in children[xxxii]. The two which are most often seen are an inability to swallow – you will know if this happens – and food aversion. The second of these is generally found to be fairly specific. For example, some adults have been identified who find it impossible to make themselves eat green vegetables[xxxiii]. They can be treated by professionals using hypnotherapy and other techniques. So, if you think that your child is showing signs of an aversion, do a quick reality-check: is it a particular type of food that he or she is avoiding or is it more general? If your little boy won't eat vegetables of any kind whatsoever, then I am afraid that is unlikely to be a food aversion because there is so much variation in what a vegetable looks, tastes and feels like. But if he only tries to avoid carrots, oranges and sweet potatoes, there may be some negative association that he has developed relating to orange food. Remember, these issues are very rare, but if you do suspect a food phobia then talk to a professional because these types of problems can become linked to more extreme eating disorders over time.

Here is a summary of the rules I have set out above.

5. Limit meals to a reasonable length.
6. Organise meals to ensure that the rejected foods are eaten.
7. Exclude disruptive influences.
8. Manage shock tactics as food refusal.

Food is Rewarding

Rule 25: reward healthy eating choices

So now you have thrown out the junk food in your house, organised mealtimes so that everyone eats the same things, proactively dealt with disruptive elements and eradicated behaviour designed to divert you from your aim. What we set out to do is threefold. You want your children to be able to choose, eat and enjoy healthy food. As adults, this will help them to continue a healthy lifestyle. They will be less likely to be overweight or to suffer illness than other people who choose or have been allowed to develop unhealthy diets.

You may feel that, by now, your children are eating and enjoying their food. I hope that what you are giving them to eat at home is healthy and – if not exemplary – at least excludes any junk. But how do you make sure they choose the healthy option all the time, when at home and away from home, and how do they get used to making this choice over and over again?

A good way to encourage sustained healthy eating is simply to reward members of the family who have chosen good things to eat. Almost subconsciously, most of you will already be doing this to some extent. Here is how.

Grace: "Hi, Dad."

Dad: "Hello, love. Did you have a good day?"

Grace: "Yes, I have got a new book to read. It's about a mouse."

Dad: "That sounds good. We'll read it at bed-time, then. What did you have for lunch today?"

Grace: " I had, um, tomatoes and carrots and beans."

Dad: "Baked beans?"

Grace: "Yes – and, um, some pizza."

Dad: "Did you have anything else?"

Grace: "A yoghourt."

Dad: "That sounds like quite a good meal. Well done for having vegetables."

This is an "actual" meal that my daughter reported that she had eaten at school one day. Obviously, young children do find it quite hard to remember exactly what they have eaten! But the important thing is that the little girl's father is saying the right things. First, he is interested in what she has eaten and, very importantly, he is telling her that she has done well to eat some vegetables.

If you want to develop healthy eating further you might try starting a family food chart and reward system. This need not be complicated: giving your children ticks on a sheet of paper for every vegetable or fruit portion eaten would work just fine. It is just a way of making healthy eating fun and gives positive feedback for doing what is good for everyone. Just ignore "bad" foods and don't give them a tick. The rationale for doing this is that it is quite hard to fit in much unhealthy stuff if you are eating plenty of the right food groups. In my family, as long as everyone is eating plenty of fruit and vegetables, some unhealthy foods can be ignored.

Rule 26: make healthy food cool

As part of the research for this book, I carried out a series of interviews with teenagers. Often seen as the most difficult age-group regarding eating habits, the children I spoke to still appeared to be pretty aware of the need to eat healthily. Most of them said that the biggest influence on what they chose to eat was their parents. The second most important factor was the information they had learned from school about what they should eat and why. All of them told me about eating "five-a-day" and all of them said they ate rather more chocolates and sweet things than they should do!

But what I found very interesting was that all of a sudden, eating at fast food outlets isn't as "cool" as it was. The teenagers I spoke to now view this type of food as the relatively poor quality meal option that it is. They used words such as "dirty", "unhealthy" and "not nice" to describe what a fast-food outlet feels like. They would all – and this was without exception – like to eat out with their families at an Italian restaurant, generally a chain such as "Pizza Express" or "Bella Pasta". With their friends, they choose cheaper options, but still prefer a sandwich to a pie from the bakers.

What this suggests is that there is some cultural change in how we, including our children, view food. The high media focus on obesity, what we eat and how much we exercise, must be having some effect.

You can "exploit" this to help ensure that your children continue to make the healthy choice through life. First of all, it is good news that children seem to listen to their parents more than we had thought. This means that your nagging is not completely pointless! There is so much that your children can read, hear and see about food and you can make sure that you share the seeing, listening and hearing. Discuss food at home – especially at mealtimes. Talk about what your children eat and what others eat. Keep a food diary and, when it is complete, use it to talk through how items of poor nutritional value can be replaced with healthier alternatives – but which are still a "cool" choice for your child.

If you are going out to a restaurant for a special treat, talk about some of the options regarding where everyone might want to go and agree which one gives the best choice of good-quality food, which each of you will be happy with.

Rule 13 (again): ignore the behaviour you do not want – do not make a fuss

In the section about rewarding children for healthy choices, I mentioned that junk food should be ignored as long as you feel your children are eating lots of the healthier types of food. If there is very little junk food in your house and you are confident that your children are eating healthy food at home and at school, it serves no real purpose to make a huge fuss if they come home from football and tell you that they had a fizzy drink and a bag of crisps after the match. Over time, and as they develop (hopefully) a more sophisticated palate, they probably will find fizzy drinks too sweet to eat and crisps too salty. They may have eaten it because it was offered by another child and they felt it would be rude not to. Or perhaps everyone else was eating the crisps, so they did it, too.

I think this approach applies to eating out, as well. Having a meal in a restaurant is a great opportunity for your children to try out new things which you may not have the time or the inclination to cook at home. They might fancy the really hot curry, the cannelloni or the lobster, followed by the sticky toffee pudding, for instance. We once took a nine year-old out with us for a meal and he chose snails as his starter! Anyway, I do not think that this is a good time to worry whether your family will be achieving its five-a-day target. Both you and your children will enjoy the experience more if they are allowed free rein to choose what they want to eat.

Rule 27: encourage and support your children to cook

The UK Government has made cookery classes compulsory for all 11- to 16-year olds. But cooking should also be something that children can get involved in at home. Many of my friends "do cooking" with their children. I popped to see a neighbour recently and we had a glass of wine each while her fourteen-year old was cooking the family meal for the evening in the background. Ever since they were very small, my children wanted to help in the kitchen and stood on chairs either side of the "island" unit, so that they could add ingredients, mix, butter dishes and do all manner of things to assist me. Obviously, this became more useful as they got older and could break an egg without it falling on the floor!

Partly the reason I did this with them was because I vividly remember my grandmother letting me watch her make all sorts of meals whenever I went to stay with her. I only know how to make things like gravy, for example, from watching her do it. And this is why I know how valuable this involved learning is for children.

Inspiring your child to cook and to be interested in food isn't only about getting them to do it. Why not take them to a restaurant where they can see the chef making the food? Pizza places are often good for this. Or take them fruit picking and make some jam with the results. If you go to the seaside, see if you can watch a catch come in and then go to a seafood restaurant for lunch or dinner. We once watched two boats full of angry-looking lobsters and crabs come up the jetty and unload at a north east coastal fishing village – the children were fascinated by this. If there is a "maize maze" near you, then they might have an eating-the-maize event which takes place when the harvest is ready. Gardens and country-house estates might have special events such as mushroom foraging or pumpkin-growing and pumpkin pie-making competitions. Village shows have a wide range of cookery classes to enter, including for children.

There are so many ways in which you can get your children to understand that cooking is part of everyday life and that they can be involved and find it an interesting experience. Lots of books are aimed specifically at children of all ages. The teenagers that I spoke to during my research were all able to tell me about the TV chefs they liked and whose cooking they thought was good. Going back to the idea of making food "cool", they clearly felt that cooking was something that everyone should do and that it could be fun

If you are going to let your offspring loose in the kitchen, I recommend that you are "on hand" for any advice or crisis that may occur the first few times. After this, you will be surprised at how quickly they become competent. It goes without saying that you should be 100% supportive of their attempts and appreciative of the outcome. Good luck.

In summary, you need to:
25. Reward healthy eating choices.
26. Make healthy food cool.
27. Encourage and support your children to cook.
You also need to continue to
13. Ignore the behaviour you do not want – do not make a fuss.

Summary

The principles behind establishing good eating habits in children from the age of about four or five onwards are very similar to those that are relevant to younger children. Try to agree any new rules that you wish to apply in advance and, whenever possible, get family members involved in getting rewards for eating healthily, in sharing ideas for meals and in cooking them.

Keep things in perspective and think carefully about how you respond to difficult behaviour, including refusing food and shock tactics. You may have to be relatively more firm and consistent than with younger children, but as long as you are clear what the rules of your house are, you should see some changes over time. Remember that children do actually listen to and are influenced by both what you say and how you behave and think about whether you need to adapt your own behaviour accordingly.

Consider how food can be rewarding for the whole family and how you can start to measure the changes that you want to see happen. Over time, everyone should be able to relax at mealtimes and the people who will benefit most are all of you. As a parent or carer, your life will be simpler and less stressful. Your children will feel happier with lots of different things to eat and I hope they will find mealtimes more interesting. I have never come across a youngster who doesn't enjoy cooking. If you can get them "into" this now, they should be competent cooks by the time they leave home. Hopefully, this will give them a happier, healthier and longer life.

This chapter has built on the previous sections of the book by introducing a number of rules aimed specifically at a slightly older age group, from the age of about four upwards. They are as shown over the page.

Rule number	The rule
Back to Proper Meals	
17	One meal, one mealtime
18	Avoid the pitfall of grazing
19	Chuck out the junk
20	Increase the range of foods that you eat
Manage Avoidance	
21	Limit meals to a reasonable length of time
22	Organise meals to ensure that the rejected foods are eaten
23	Exclude disruptive influences
24	Manage shock tactics as food refusal
Food is Rewarding	
25	Reward healthy eating choices
26	Make healthy food cool
13 (again)	Ignore the behaviour you do not want – do not make a fuss
27	Encourage and support your children to cook

6 A HEALTHY DIET

If you are in a state of panic about what a balanced diet really should be, or if you think you know what healthy food is, but you are not sure whether baked beans are good or bad, then please sit down for half an hour and read through this brief outline. I have checked the facts in this chapter out with a qualified clinical nutritionist, so you can be sure they are current and accurate.

Take in and absorb the messages and just make sure that you have a clear idea in your mind about how these translate into meals in your house. For example, if you need to provide at least five portions of fruit and vegetables each day, you might say to yourself, "I need to give the children one glass of juice or smoothie for breakfast, an apple, banana or pear for a snack, one vegetable or salad item at lunchtime and two vegetables (frozen, fresh or raw) or one vegetable and one fruit at teatime." Breaking the requirements down in this way make healthy eating choices seem far less daunting. Menu planning is also a good way to take some of the stress out of meal preparation. You can then plan in two meals each week with oily fish, for instance. One might be sardines and tomatoes on toast for tea and one might be baked salmon fillets for a weekend meal. And what you cook or prepare does not need to be complicated or ambitious to tick the balanced diet boxes.

Basic nutrition guidelines

Good sources of clear information about what you should be eating, if you want more detail than I have given below, are the Food Standards Agency via their Eat Well website (www.eatwell.gov.uk) and the British Nutrition Foundation (www.nutrition.org.uk).

The components of a balanced diet are made up of four food groups:

- Cereals, bread and potatoes
- Fruit and vegetables
- Milk and dairy foods and
- Meat, fish, pulses and other alternatives.

Straight away you will have noticed that there is no food group for things including cakes, biscuits and crisps. The truth is that no one needs fatty, sugary food in their diet – they are not a requirement for good health and for living. They are not included in the Government's guidance or the British Medical Association's, or the British Heart Foundation's because they are not necessary. You and your children can still eat them. But you shouldn't be eating them instead of one of the other food groups. What this means is that a snack between meals should never be just a packet of crisps or a couple of biscuits. Add a piece of fruit or a handful of raisins or offer these on their own and you will be doing your children a big favour in the aim to achieve that five-a-day target.

What about the other food groups? Let's start with fruit and vegetables. You should eat *at least* (note - that says "at least" – not "only") five portions of these per day. You can count frozen, tinned and dried versions, as well as fresh fruit and vegetables. You can also include one glass of fruit juice (three glasses still counts as just one, by the way). Baked beans can be counted once, too. Potatoes, including sweet potatoes, don't count in this group. Most people do not eat enough fruit and vegetables.

Similarly, most of us don't eat enough cereal and other starchy carbohydrates such as pasta, rice, oats, noodles, polenta (cornmeal) etc. If you want to be really healthy, you should eat wholegrain/wholemeal versions. Eating too much refined food (white versions of bread, pasta, etc) can result in your body being unable to metabolise the energy within it, if it is not balanced by other key food components. The idea is that the main constituent of a meal should be this food group, supported by plenty of fruit and vegetables, plus a reasonable proportion of dairy and meat or fish – type foods. About one-third of what you eat should be foods from this group. They are the prime source of energy for our bodies.

You should eat two or three servings per day of dairy products, including in teas and coffees. But you have to be careful because they are generally quite fatty. So, even if you buy a low-fat version of something, you still need to be aware that they came from a high-fat starting point and probably remain relatively high in fat. For this reason, butter and cream are not in this food group. Be aware that children under the age of five need more fat than adults and older children. You can give them full-fat yoghurt, milk and so on.

A similar group of foods are meat, fish and alternatives, which can be fresh, frozen or canned. Some of these can be high in fat, so they need to be balanced or minimised. As with all foods, how you cook it will affect the amount of fat it contains. Meat and fish are high in protein, which is why they, or meat-free alternatives, are needed in our diet. But many people eat far too much red meat and not enough of the other options, such as oily fish. Recent evidence from the World Cancer Research Fund suggests that we should limit our intake of red meat to a maximum of 500 grammes per week and avoid processed meats altogether. This food group also includes poultry, fish and eggs as well as nuts, tofu, beans and lentils. You need to eat one or two portions each day of these types of foods.

Finally, most people eat too many fatty and sugary foods. This is surely part of our culture and forms part of our up-bringing. But almost all of us eat too much butter, or chocolate, or the odd bag of crisps. Your fat requirements are almost certainly covered by the other things you eat, so you really don't need any of these foods. I don't think anyone is suggesting that no-one should ever eat these types of food, but it is probably best for your children to avoid them as snacks and only eat them as part of a main meal which has the other food groups in balance.

How you cook food

You probably already know that it is not a good idea to fry food. However healthy the constituents of a meal, frying it basically adds unnecessary fat to what you are eating. This and other forms of cooking at high temperatures – grilling and roasting – have a particular effect on certain fats, which nutritionists and scientists are concerned about. Trans fats are a by-product of heating. When polyunsaturated oils are heated they twist and re-form into new compounds. These block the body's absorption of essential amino acids, including important ones such as Omega 3. Saturated fats like olive and rapeseed oil, butter and goose fat are more stable at high temperatures and therefore better for us – even though we need to be careful not to eat too much of any fats overall.

Something about salt.

Too much salt is bad for you because it increases your risk of stroke and heart disease. About 75% of the salt in the diet of people across the UK comes from processed foods. So if, as a family, you buy and consume a lot of pre-prepared and ready meals, including things like oven-ready fish, sauces in jars, pizzas and so on, you should be aware that you are probably eating more than enough salt in those foods and you certainly should not be adding any more while cooking or at the table. You may actually be eating too much salt and should think about whether to choose low-salt options in future. However, the Government, through the Food Standards Agency, has been working with the food industry to reduce salt levels, which will help over time.
Your children should be eating very little salt:

- Between 4 and 6 years – up to 3 grammes per day
- Between 7 and 10 years up to 5 grammes per day
- From 11 years – up to 6 grammes per day.

The maximum recommended amount for adults is about 7 grammes per day. The basic advice is not to add salt to children's food at all.

Children's nutrition

In general, children should keep to the balance of food outlined above. However, there are some variations in what they need for health, which derive from the fact that they are growing and need more of both energy-giving and specific nutrient-providing foods than adults do.

Before the age of six months, current advice is that babies should be given milk (breast or formula) alone, to meet their nutritional requirements. You should talk to your GP or health visitor if you want more information about feeding before this age.

After weaning and up to the age of around three years, children need more energy. Their diets need to be "energy-dense". This means plenty of all the four food groups listed, plus full fat milk. From this age on, though, we still need to make sure that children are eating at least five portions of fruit and vegetables every day.

From the age of five, children no longer need to consume full-fat milk. They can drink semi-skimmed or skimmed milk. Through the remainder of childhood, the energy and protein requirements of children increase. This means they need to eat more of the foods which provide these. They also need to continue eating a balance of fruit and vegetables which will maintain the variety of vitamins and minerals that their bodies need. Once girls start their periods, they have a higher requirement of iron than boys do. From the age of about 15, all children need a range of vitamins and minerals for healthy development and these should all be provided by a balanced diet. However, this is also an age where growth of bones is rapid, so there is still a need for plenty of calcium in your children's diets.

Find ideas for healthy family meals

I am not going to set out here how to cook fabulous healthy meals for a family of four. There are plenty of other books which can help with that. There are quite a few books which are aimed at people who want to be able to produce a meal in under half-an-hour, under twenty minutes or under fifteen, if you are short of time. There is a huge wealth of recipe information on the internet, as well.

When thinking about the five-a-day rule, don't forget that there are lots of alternatives to freshly-prepared and cooked fruit and vegetables – tins, frozen and dried versions. The retailers are gearing their product ranges to help us in this area, as well – labelling often shows how much is equal to a portion, or how many portions are contained in a packet.

Some meals you can cheat at by buying some or all of the components ready-made. For example, you can buy good-quality sauces and soups in supermarkets, which are made with fresh ingredients. But remember that the more you cook yourself, the less likely you are to be eating too much salt, sugar and fat. Remember also that a good way to reduce the load on the cook is to make double quantities where possible and to freeze half for later.

If you would like ideas for children's lunch-boxes, then the Eat Well website mentioned above is a good place to start.

Summary

My guess is that most people nowadays have some understanding of the basics of nutrition. Hopefully, this final chapter has clarified any broad queries you may have. If it has not, do check out the websites I have mentioned. They also include menus, recipes and ideas for healthy eating – all of which should inspire you and your family to cook rewarding healthy meals. Then, you need to get on with the business of eating it all up.

Did you like it?

What did you think of "Eat It All Up?" Is it useful, would you recommend it? Would you like more information?

Please let me know, by going to my website:

www.eatitallup.com

LIST OF REFERENCES

[i] The research for this was carried out by L.A. Proos in 1993: "Anthropometry in adolescence – secular trends, adoption, ethnic and environmental differences", published in *Hormone Research*, vol 39, pp 18-24.

[ii] From the Health Survey for England, 2009, available on the department of health's website (www.dh.gov.uk).

[iii] National Diet and Nutrition Survey; Headline results from the Rolling Programme (2008/9-2009/10), available on the department of health's website, as above.

[iv] From the Health Survey for England, statistical data from 2006 to 2009, available on the department of health's website, as above.

[v] "The pack-a-day habit threatening our kids' health", 22 September 2006. Part of the Food4Thought campaign launched by the British Heart Foundation in 2006.

[vi] House of Commons Health Committee (2004) *Obesity, third report of session 2003-04, Volume 1*. London: The Stationery Office.

[vii] Dr Sam Everington and Partners, reported in, *Preventing Childhood Obesity*, BMA, June 2005, London.

[viii] From the National Diet and Nutrition Survey: Children aged 1½ to 4½ years. Volume 1: Report of the Diet and Nutrition Survey. OPCS. Compiled by J.R.Gregory, D.L. Collins, P.S.W. Davies, J.M. Hughes and P.C. Clarke and published in 1995 by HMSO, London

[ix] As reported, for example, by Epstein et al (1994) "Effects of mastery criteria and contingent reinforcement for family-based child weight control", in *Addictive Behaviours*, 19, 135-145.

[x] Joanna Blythman, *Bad Food Britain: How a Nation Ruined its Appetite,* 2006, London, Fourth Estate.

[xi] This was reported to the Department of Health in 1990, by Day.

[xii] Reported by Asthma UK in their website section on diet and food. www.asthma.org.uk.

[xiii] The British Medical Association's excellent paper produced by their Board of Science. *Preventing Childhood Obesity*, BMA, June 2005, London.

[xiv] International Obesity TaskForce (2004) *Obesity in children and young people, a crisis in public health.* www.iotf.org. Contact: childhood@iotf.org

[xv] Latner JD. & Stunkard AJ (2003) Getting worse: the stigmatization of obese children. *Obesity Research.* **11(3):** 452-6.

[xvi] These findings were reported by S.C. Gortmaker et al (1993) in "The social and economic consequences of overweight in adolescence and young adulthood": *New England Journal of Medicine*, 329, 1008-1012.

[xvii] From the Channel 4 website, Jamie Oliver's experience of making the programme *"Jamie's School Dinners"*. www.channel4.com.

[xviii] This was reported across the national press during June and July 2006, for example on the BBC News website, 21 July 2006, *Cadbury's "linked" to salmonella"*.

[xix] From the Food Standards Agency website: www.food.gov.uk.

[xx] A team from Newcastle General Hospital, led by Dr Andrew Cant, carried out this research, which was published in the *Archives of Disease in Childhood* and reported by the BBC on 25 March 2002. www.bbc.co.uk.

[xxi] This is reported in *The Independent*, 28 November 2005, and references the most recent research, carried out by Julie Mennella of the Monell Institute in Philadelphia.

[xxii] Annabel Karmel is a well-known author in this area. Examples include her *New Complete Baby and Toddler Meal Planner,* Ebury Press, published in 2008.

[xxiii] Joanna Blythman, *Bad Food Britain: How a Nation Ruined its Appetite,* 2006, London, Fourth Estate.

[xxiv] This research was carried out by Birch et al, 1991, "The variability of young children's energy intake", *NewEngland Journal of Medicine,* 324, pp232-235.

[xxv] Mostly carried out by Isobel Contento at the Columbia University's Teachers' College.

[xxvi] The research was led by Lucy Cooke on behalf of Cancer Research UK and published in *Public Health Nutrition*, 7 (2). It was the subject of a press release: 7 March 2004. *"Parents need to set example by eating more fruit and veg"*, included on the CRUK website.

[xxvii] Jamie's School Dinners was shown on Channel 4 during 2004 and led to a dramatic improvement in the range of healthy food options available to children for school lunches.

[xxviii] One example of research in this area is Birch, L.L. and Fisher, J.A. in "Appetite and Eating Behaviour in Children", *Pediatrics Clinics of North America*, 1995, 42, pp931-953.

[xxix] The impact of social environment is established by Birch, L.L., Zimmerman, S. and Hind, H, "The Influence of Social-Affective Context on Preschool Children's Food Preferences", *Child Development*, 1980, 51, pp856-861.

[xxx] Reported by the Eating Disorders Unit of the Institute of Child Health at University College London. The web address is: www.ich.ucl.ac.uk/factsheets/families and search for Eating Disorders.

[xxxi] Explained in Sullivan, S.A. and Birch, L.L., "Pass the Sugar, Pass the Salt; Experience Dictates Preference", *Developmental Psychology,* 1990, 26, pp546-551.

[xxxii] See information from The Eating Disorders Unit of the Institute of Child Health at University College London. www.ich.ucl.ac.uk/factsheets/families and search for Eating Disorders.

[xxxiii] This was reported, for example, in an article in the Telegraph on 7 October 2006.

ABOUT THE AUTHOR

Louise Brennan wanted to be a journalist when she was growing up. Instead, she went to university, got a degree in Psychology and went to work in the National Health Service for eight years. Deciding she couldn't change the world from there she went on to be a management consultant, advising businesses on strategy. After her children were born, she realised she still hadn't changed the world. However, she did notice that lots of her friends' children didn't eat what they were given....whereas hers did.

Louise lives in the Yorkshire Dales with her husband, two children and around thirteen chickens. As well as this book, she has written a number of articles on children's eating habits for The Yorkshire Post.

Made in the USA
Charleston, SC
29 June 2012